Missing Kali

Also by Kali Rae Wheeler

Losing Kali
Finding Kali

BOOK 3 OF THE FINDING KALI TRILOGY

Missing Kali

Moving to LA, Rx Side Effects Include
Navigating College in a Pharmaceutical Blackout

Kali Rae Wheeler

Copyright 2017 © Kali Rae Wheeler. All rights reserved. No part of this book may be reproduced in any form or by any electronic or mechanical means, including information storage and retrieval systems, without written permission from the author, except in the case of a reviewer, who may quote brief passages embedded in critical articles or in a review.

Trademarked names appear throughout this book. Rather than use a trademark symbol with every occurrence of a trademarked name, names are used in an editorial fashion, with no intention of infringement of the respective owner's trademark.

The information in this book is distributed on an "as is" basis, without warranty. Although every precaution has been taken in the preparation of this work, neither the author nor the publisher shall have any liability to any person or entity with respect to any loss or damage caused or alleged to be caused directly or indirectly by the information contained in this book.

I have tried to recreate events, locales and conversations from my memories of them. In order to maintain their anonymity in some instances I have changed the names of individuals and places, I may have changed some identifying characteristics and details such as physical properties, occupations and places of residence.

ISBN: 978-1629670973

Library of Congress Control Number: 2017942526

This book is dedicated to the people struggling with either a mental disorder or a pseudo-mental disorder fueled by Big Pharma, abuse, or trauma, and to anyone who's ever been a victim of sexual assault or sexual misconduct in the workplace and to any soul who's been struck by the increase in mass shootings around the nation and our world.

We are all in this together.

Love and light to you.

XO, Kali Rae

To the gritty ones, the loyal, the optimists by necessity, here's to the ones who have been tested the most:

"I love those who can smile in trouble, who can gather strength from distress, and grow brave by reflection. 'Tis the business of little minds to shrink, but they whose heart is firm, and whose conscience approves their conduct, will pursue their principles unto death." Leonardo Da Vinci

Contents

PREFACE	III
THANK YOU	V
INTRODUCTION	VI
AUTHOR'S NOTE	IX
FOREWORD	XIII
ABBREVIATIONS AND TERMS	XV
LIST OF DOCTORS	XVIII
1 FROM THE COAST TO THE HILLS	1
...BUT FIRST, LEXAPRO...	2
A TASTE OF FIASCHETTI'S PRESCRIBING HX	4
THE LEATHER JOURNAL: THE CITY OF ANGELS	5
August 22, 2009	*6*
August 23, 2009	*7*
AARON "SHOWS ME AROUND LA"	8
NO WAY OUT, CUTTING TIES	11
CLINGING TO HOME	13
DANE EDWARDS: THE DICK ACROSS THE HALL	16
THE LEATHER JOURNAL: INITIATION INTO THE CITY	18
August 27, 2009	*19*
August 31, 2009	*21*
OVERPRESCRIBING SERIOUSLY DANGEROUS MEDICATIONS	24
TAKING CARE OF MY HEALTH, A PERSONAL TRAINER	25
FORCING A MILKSHAKE; CONTROL FREAK CLUES	28
AN ALARMING PHONE CALL	31
UNEXPECTED GAME OF RUSSIAN ROULETTE	34
STACKED LESIONS	37
THE LEATHER JOURNAL: NEGLECTED	40
November 15, 2009	*41*
MISSING JAXX, JAY GATSBY	42
BACK IN HIS ATMOSPHERE	44
THE CITY OF STARS	46
THE RED CAP	48
TRIALS WITH GATSBY	50
THE NIGHT IS YOUNG	53
AUTOPILOT INTO THE GHETTO	55
THE WRITING ON THE WALL	57

Petiole: January 2010 — 60
LOSING CONTROL — 62
A FISH OUTTA WATER — 66
THE SERENITY JOURNAL — 73
   January 15, 2010 — 74
   January 21, 2010 — 76
   January 22, 2010 — 77
   January 23, 2010 — 78
THE DOCTOR'S BEACH HOUSE — 79
ULTRAM — 83
   January 30, 2010 — 85
   Pure Whites: January 2010 — 87
   Black Or White: February 8, 2010 — 89
NCPD: THE COURAGE TO SPEAK UP — 90
TELLING MY STORY — 93
HE LAUGHS AT MY JOKES, DRIVES, AND SUPPORTS EVERYTHING I DO AND SAY/ I DON'T HAVE TIME TO SAY NO TO THAT — 96
"LET'S GET A PUPPY" — 98
DON'T F*** WITH MY BROTHER — 102
DR. FIASCHETTI, M.D. (PSYCHIATRIST) — 105
FOOLED: THIS DEFINITELY ISN'T DAVE MATTHEWS. — 108
"PLEASE RECOUNT THOSE" — 111
THE SERENITY JOURNAL: IN NOT SO SERENE TIMES — 113
   Writing to You from Sunny, Santa Barbara, California — 114
   June 19, 2010 — 115
   We Could: June 20, 2010 — 116
RIFAMPIN: NIGHT TERRORS, NEAR-PSYCHOSIS, DEMENTIA — 118
BREAKING UP/THE BAYFRONT PROPOSAL — 123
THE SERENITY JOURNAL: NO MEMORIES, NO CRY — 125
   June 29th, 2010: — 126
   A List of Names — 127
   June 30, 2010 — 128
   July 1, 2010 — 131
   July 2, 2010 — 132
   Those Eyes — 133
   July 6, 2010 — 134
   July 7, 2010 — 135
   July 8, 2010 — 136
   July 10, 2010 — 137
   Enough: July 15, 2010 — 138
   July 16, 2010 — 139
   Stolen: July 17, 2010 — 140
   July 19, 2010 — 142

Battlefield: July 19, 2010	*143*
Think You In: July 19, 2010	*144*
July 24, 2010	*145*
July 30, 2010	*148*
July 30, 2010	*149*
July 31, 2010	*150*
I Don't Wanna Remember: July 31, 2010	*151*
I Left: July 31, 2010	*152*
July 31, 2010	*153*
August 1, 2010	*154*
Returning the Ring	*155*

2 BACK TO THE CITY, CLASSES IN THE HILLS — 156

NOT A FASHION VIRGIN	157
A CORPORATE FASHION INTERNSHIP	159
THE PHOTOG	162
ALL HEROIN, NOT CHIC	165
August 29, 2010	*167*
MIKAH	168
September 6, 2010	*170*
POEMS FROM A NEW/THE SAME PLACE: FALL 2010	171
Cold: September 7, 2010	*172*
Sometimes I Wish: September 9, 2010	*173*
Suck It Up: September 9, 2010	*174*
September 10, 2010	*175*
Her Own Space: October 3, 2010	*176*
The Effects of Studying for an Exam Given by Professor Divine: Fall 2010	
	178
Falling Faster: Fall 2010	*179*
Galveston Falling Away: Fall 2010	*180*
I Love You, Maybe: Fall 2010	*181*
Chains: Fall 2010	*182*
Am I Lost or Was I Left: Fall 2010	*183*
Fractured Planet: Fall 2010	*185*
Your Worst Enemy: Fall 2010	*186*
Da Vinci's Muse: Fall 2010	*187*
What to Make of It All: November 25, 2010	*188*
DR. BRAUN	189
Truck Driver, December 19, 2010	*202*
THE AUDITION	204
THE FISH TANK INCIDENT	206
Beneath a Steamer: January 23, 2011	*214*
9-1-1; THINGS ESCALATE QUICKLY	219
MEETING THE NEIGHBORS	236

WANDERING INTO A FRAT HOUSE	238
The Fraternal Instincts: Spring 2011	*240*
THROUGH THE WINDOW	242
A Paramedic's Mistake: Spring 2011	*249*
MAMMOTH	253
HIS EYES: LAPSES PART 1	258
DRIVING TO GET STELLA: LAPSES PART 2	262
Till Morning's Light: Spring 2011	*265*
THE ACCIDENT	267
GETTING TO TRIAGE	271
WHAT FUCKING FLOOR?!	273
A Poem for Dr. Braun: April 23, 2011	*288*
A FRIENDLY NEUROLOGIST	289
Mistress Overcome: Spring 2011	*293*
INTERLUDE: ALL MY FRIENDS ARE DOCTORS	295
DRUGGED BY THE DJ...FOR MY BIRTHDAY	296
Mr. Wrong: Spring 2011	*300*
MOVING & PAINT THERAPY	302
Angel: Spring 2011	*305*
Fan-Mail Repetition	*310*
THE VIBES CHANGED	311
A STARTER PACK TO HELL: SAVELLA	314
THE POET	315
JASPER IN LOS FLORES	317
BRENT IS ON DRUGS, OR HE WAS...	320
BRENT IS NUTS, FOR REAL	325
UNDER THE LIGHTS:...CAMERA, ACTION!	327
September 3, 2011: Species	*330*

3. EPILOGUE NOT ONLY ARE MY DOCTORS FAMOUS (*LOSING KALI* JOKE), SO ARE MY ATTACKERS   331
   AARON'S ARTICLE   332
   JASON'S ARTICLE   335

AFTERWORD   337
   SIDE EFFECTS INCLUDE DEATH   338
   THE FACTS ABOUT PHARMACEUTICALS, EDUCATE YOURSELF   341
   MANIPULATING THE PATIENTS   343

APPENDICES   346
   APPENDIX A   347
   APPENDIX B   350
   APPENDIX C   351
   APPENDIX D   352
   APPENDIX E   354

APPENDIX F	355
APPENDIX G	356
APPENDIX H	358
APPENDIX I	361
APPENDIX J	364
APPENDIX K	365
APPENDIX L	366
APPENDIX M	367
APPENDIX N	369
APPENDIX O	371
APPENDIX P	372
APPENDIX Q	373
APPENDIX R	374
APPENDIX S	375
APPENDIX T	376
APPENDIX U	378
APPENDIX V	380
APPENDIX W	383
APPENDIX Y	385
APPENDIX X	386
GLOSSARY OF USEFUL TERMS	**387**
REFERENCES	**388**
THANK YOU	**396**

Missing Kali

Preface

[DISCLAMER: Same Info as *Losing Kali*]

Seven years from the time my pharmaceutical hell commenced, I found myself in a frenzied search for answers. I was past the point of realizing what had happened to me and was now out for justice. It was time to become the detective of my past and place the pieces of this catastrophic jigsaw puzzle back together.

I needed to collect information outside of my experiences. I found myself reeling from the pain surfacing from all the self-excavation. I needed the inspiration to press forward, to continue past how much I wanted to pull my hair out and burn the doctors' records.

I found a few documentaries while working late night in the recording studio, which provided a spark of perseverance and the validity to continue climbing the mountain toward the summit. A clear pattern was emerging; the things I experienced were not unique to me; they were plaguing the nation, even if it was behind closed doors. There was a real bad ass monster that I needed to slay for the rest of us. One documentary in particular, *Boy Interrupted* (Perry 2009) clarified a critical concept and emblazoned it into my mind.

The documentary is about a teenage boy who suffered from bipolar disorder. He showed signs as early as two years old. He had dramatic mood swings where he said violent things. He would isolate himself. He would throw tantrums. All the typical mental illness checkmarks were there. He was also very well-liked and had many friends.

After weaning himself off his prescriptions due to their adverse side effects; feeling tired, numb, headachy, etc., that he had reportedly (by parents, teachers, and friends) been doing so well on, he tragically took his own life.

What shook me to the core was what he had written on his laptop just moments before. He wrote of the universal emotions that plague the process of growing up. They were emotions that I had documented clearly, but more important, remembered clearly, and felt so profoundly. The catch is that I reported feeling these things more powerfully while under the influence of psychotropic drugs.

My lack of self-awareness and inability to control impulses came out of thin air. I might have felt the same things no matter what, but when I was on the drugs, my desire to act was tangible. Many times I felt like I was being drawn to the edge of the cliff or taunted by the pill bottle to take more. I can still, to this day, remember the unmistakable surge of adrenaline that accompanied these feelings. It was animalistic: the feeling similar to sprinting the last quarter-mile of a 5k marathon using some strength and speed I never knew I had.

The impulses were often so intense that I had to have my best friend Tessa babysit me, or at least stay on the phone with me until they passed. I often pondered how much time it would take to break away from whoever I was with and jump off the nearest bridge. Each time I'd have this intense drive to kill myself. But thoughts of being disabled instead of killed by the fall plagued me. If I was pondering using pills, I would worry that I would end up a vegetable, which would put even more of a burden on my parents. The thoughts that held me back were the possibility that the attempt would not produce fatal results.

I would come to find years later, that not only was the impulse to take my life stronger while I was under the influence of prescription drugs, the ideations themselves might have been a direct result of the drugs themselves.

By miracle, I am alive today to tell you that a mentally ill, chemically imbalanced person becomes balanced when given the right chemicals and therefore, he steps back from the ledge.

A chemically stable, but emotionally unstable teenager given the same brain-altering drugs becomes chemically imbalanced on top of everything else going on in a growing brain, and therefore, he or she is propelled toward the ledge. It is a biochemical equation; imbalanced, apt to jump, balanced naturally but put into a state of artificial imbalance, apt to jump. The latter is possibly even more dangerous than the former. It all depends upon the strength of the imbalance, whether it be biological or pharmaceutical, the equation doesn't change

Thank You

Thank you, Dad, for the support through thick and thin, for helping me through every crisis I encountered during the missing years and after. You've never stopped being my guardian in disguise, sometimes even working behind the scenes.

Thank you, Mom, for your constant support and enthusiasm. Without you I would not be here today, I am sure of that. Connected always, even when we wish we could disconnect. I don't hate it…

Thank you to my brother for working behind the scenes to help me out even when I wasn't able to understand your support. And for sending me music to get me through the hardest times…

Thank you to my sister for always testing me and for always loving me. Thank you for being you. You are a boss.

Thank you, Grandma. I am so lucky to know you. Thank you for not only supporting me, but inspiring me, pushing me and basically being the entire reason any of these books were released from my nervous fingers.

Introduction

It's dull today.

The sky is more gray than ever. And I've been in a rut. All the yoga and meditation and the Vitamix I used to do my one-week juice cleanse seemed less inspiring than usual. Right now I am afraid to move. I want to disappear and I'm not sure why this happens right at the exact time I need to step up to the plate.

I'm constantly searching for a better way to feel, a better way to live. I am obsessed with finding bliss, and in the everyday, I'm obsessed with feeling better. And I haven't been feeling better lately. No matter what I try.

Today I decided to go back to my old stomping grounds. The place where I experienced so much pain and so much insanity.

I lost my mind and wrote about it. Then argued that my poem wasn't about me as I read it aloud to our small group of about a dozen creative writing/poetry English majors.

And today, I walked through my university's library only to find that the environment that used to work for me so late at night doesn't lift me out of the place I can't be in order to continue writing this. So I meandered out of Powell Library, paranoid that I look too old to be back here now, or maybe not, which is also a thing.

And I coincidentally found my place under the same stone steps I fell down when I was doing my final project for my final class at UCLA.

I've been down. It might have something to do with the fact that everything I thought I knew and everything I thought other people were to me, have been incorrect. And I've spent the year trying to sort that out.

I want to preface this second book of the Finding Kali series with a statement about vulnerability and the power it holds. If no one ever reads this book, I will have written about this epidemic in a voice I am actually pretty much afraid of. But there is power in the fear and in the vulnerability and there certainly is power in telling my story.

If you haven't read the first book of the series, *Losing Kali*, I recommend you do that before reading this one, not just to have the basis for understanding the insanity to follow, but because it presents the quintessential and fundamental issues and tells a completely different act within the same play.

For you rebels out there who want to skip to the second book, here's a short synopsis:

In Book 1, *Losing Kali*, Kali falls into the hands of negligent doctors. After an adverse reaction to Prozac, thoughtlessly prescribed to improve the pains of growing up, Kali gets strapped into a roller coaster of different mood stabilizers, anticonvulsants fibromyalgia drugs, migraine medications, you name it, they prescribed it.

After upping the dosage tremendously until it is almost six times what is was to begin with, Kali acts manic and Dr. Scott, Kali's primary care physician and trusted doctor, opposing Kali's mother and her gut instinct (Kali had zero mental or emotional issues growing up) diagnoses Kali as bipolar. The diagnosis of manic depression leads to psychotropic medications that take Kali out of her mind and into a very scary reality.

As a result of the continually shifting cocktail of medications, Kali is diagnosed with and medicated for such maladies as interstitial cystitis, fibromyalgia, chronic fatigue syndrome, generalized anxiety disorder, depression, ADHD, ADD, posttraumatic stress syndrome; the list goes on and on. Every time Kali is prescribed a new drug to fix the "imbalance," another layer of craziness emerges.

After a stint in rehab for an eating disorder, Kali is shoved into more and more specialists' offices, more and more money and time are thrown at the problem because nobody knows what to do.

A few psychiatrists and therapists later, Kali is still being taken on and off drugs that are extremely dangerous when mixed with adolescent chemistry, Now, however, Kali has a few diagnoses to list when she fills out intake forms and a long history of different psychotropic, benzodiazepines, fibromyalgia drugs, antidepressants, mood stabilizers, migraine treatments, and antibiotics to list on the side that asks for medicines to which she reacts adversely.

In Book 1, Kali encounters some of the very prolific issues plaguing our country at the current time, including physical and emotional abuse, sexual assault, prescription drug abuse, and the suicidal thoughts, behavior and actions caused by these medications. Kali becomes the living example of how one chink in the chain, the pharmaceutical industry and its influence on modern day medicine in this case, can cause devastating damage to every single part of the chain.

By some miracle, Kali is accepted into a top university, but this means she will be moving away from her doctors (who are killing her, but she now needs them nonetheless) and from her safe haven.

Her move to Los Angeles becomes more of a battle than anything else. Having grown up in a very sheltered community, and as a trusting young girl with zero skill at reading people, thanks to the medications, coupled with almost no impulse control, Kali walks, or rather runs, into a living hell.

If *Losing Kali* is the foundation and then the earthquake that cracks the foundation and splinters it in certain areas, *Missing Kali* is the resulting tsunami.

P.S. I left my original writings, journey scribblings and poetry, in the way I left them, so as to illustrate and preserve my mental state at the time.
.

Author's Note

[DISCLAIMER: same note as Books 1 & 2)
In the process of writing this second book of three in the "Finding Kali" series, I dug into every place I could imagine.

I compiled the journals I had meticulously kept since the invention of the gel pen. I retrieved hard copies of all of my medical records from more than a dozen different sources: doctors, therapists, hospitals, and all the different departments of medicine at the university I attended.

I scoured emails, class assignments from middle school all the way up until my last classes before receiving my B.A. and the scribblings in the margins of my notes from engineering school after that.

I searched obsessively through old social media outlets, not only to find specific dates but to reread painful conversations and find the facts amongst all the feelings. The Facebook messages were some of the worst. I'd since deactivated that account. In reactivating it, I was able to look with a microscope at the random pilings of memories and mishaps.

I typed out each and every one of the journal entries and transcribed the medical records, keepsakes, and notes written by lovers, letters from Grandma, birthday cards, everything. I needed everything I could find, no matter how painful, so that I could to place myself exactly where I had been when things occurred.

I crafted timeline after timeline, linking the medical records and notes, cross-referencing the social media conversations, photographs, and even essays written in class to coinciding events in my life.

I sorted the array of memories in piles by year, then meticulously by month and then even by day in some cases. I had to see things right next to one another, in physical form, to believe that these events happened the way that they did. I couldn't second guess cold hard facts.

For the last couple of books, especially, I retraced my steps back to the actual locations where certain events took place. Sometimes this happened by accident, like today, when I drove past the now redone brick wall I demolished when I first moved to Los Angeles, after applying for a job at that same place under the influence of Lexapro. Other times, I intentionally took a trip into the same places where my life had changed. And it took my breath away more times than I could count.

"It's okay," I would repeat to myself, transported emotionally back to the space in time that held the pain. Sometimes I got lost in the psychological trip of everything. I found myself experiencing the intense depression I used to feel, desperate to grasp on to something that wasn't shifting out from under me. It would take a full night's sleep to remember the power of shifting mindsets and the fact that we create our own realities.

Some memories came as flashbacks at places I frequent now and associate with a completely different life. The places themselves haven't changed at all, yet I hardly recognized them. I get whiplashed with the old emotions and events that transpired there.

I struggled with anger I felt toward a broken system. But also anger with myself for not doing this sooner or not realizing my own worth and getting out of situations before the exit disappeared altogether. And I spent some days mad at others and at the ways we treat each other so differently on this planet even although we are all made up of the same matter.

Having placed pieces of a sometimes intentionally forgotten puzzle back in order, I held my breath and questioned family members to get a full perspective. These were not fun conversations.

I am very auditory and often remember events solely from words exchanged. I crafted dialogue from what I remembered.

Certain people are excluded from the final book to ensure that I portray only the essential characters in getting this message across to you, the reader.

All names of individuals involved (including doctors) have been changed to protect their privacy. At certain times, specific attributes and locations have been changed to preserve the integrity of the individuals and their families.

My goal for this book has nothing to do with pointing fingers certain people. That will do no good in this situation. My goal is to shed light on an issue that is plaguing us all. We are all in this together, and as one we need to come together and fix this.

I did many hours of research on the effects of pharmaceuticals on our population, pulling from posts on discussion boards as well as articles in medical journals, medical websites, news broadcasts and even the local newspaper.

I did not include these articles in this book in order to preserve the anonymity of the people involved. By directly injecting these stories, I felt it would be overstepping my bounds into a territory that I do not need to cross to tell my story.

Lastly, the Internet searches I performed to locate some of the uniquely corrupt individuals I encountered, brought about an array of incredibly scary results.

However, with much thought, I decided that these, some of whom were even convicted criminals, deserve the right to privacy, and so I held fast to the notion that this is not a book to "out" specific parties, but rather to shed light on a terrible epidemic.

What I can say is that several doctors, as well as people and situations on this harrowing journey, have not only been brought to the of the attention of the general public, but to justice. And some of the large-scale problems I encountered have recently been the topics of news specials and in a few cases, sections of late-night comedy shows.

In order to see the beauty in something, you must stand at a distance and see it from a new angle before returning, whether that takes moments or years.

To fully immerse yourself in a message, you must let it reveal itself in its own time. If you are unable to pull yourself away, unable to hold something loosely, you will never be able to embrace it appropriately and therefore; you do not deserve its beauty. You do not recognize the work for what it is, but rather what you see in it. You are only then appreciating yourself: your perception.

If you can't let go and watch something flourish without you, you do not belong in its airspace. Once you detach, you will finally decipher the things you thought were so simple. You might unlock meanings that, until now, remained hidden from you, or new pathways that can now be treasured. You discover new reasons for being a part of this person or this message's life.

The ability to watch a piece of art draw the attention of others, to stimulate a reaction in another's mind and activate some latent memory crucial for this new person's step forward in life, that is brilliance.

In this spirit, I'm stepping back and letting go in the hope that I can save someone else from going through what I went through.

So, here it is.

Namaste.

Kali Rae

Foreword

When I first started diving back into all the places I had hidden deep in the vault that held "the missing years," I had a lot of trouble separating the present from the past. For instance, when a new artist would come into the recording studio,* I would be caught up in the emotions of the past and I wouldn't be able to answer simple questions in the present.

I shut myself up so very tight that everything was a secret. Watching the patterns of the past, I decided that I didn't want to create any more of the persona that was me. I didn't want to leave any trail behind me. I wanted to disappear. Slowly, I have found that hiding isn't fulfilling, and trying to erase every footprint behind you before stepping forward is a complete waste of time.

Becoming smaller does not build anybody else up. And speaking more softly, does not bother people less. Erasing myself from every person and situation does not rewrite history, and hiding not to make a mistake does not help anybody.

We are all put on this planet to make mistakes, learn, fall, get up, try again, and repeat. We are on a Hero's Journey.

All those years ago, in that leather journal, I promised myself I would never give up and so many times during my life I have stopped a negative pattern of thinking by remembering that promise.

---

* I worked at a very prominent record label's recording studio as an audio engineer

I'd like for you to make a promise to yourself. Once you think of a promise, I need you to write it down somewhere: write it on the page, write it on your hand, just write it down.

It is only through living that we gain the strength to conquer our deepest fears.

Dear Life,
Bring it on.
XO Kali Rae

Abbreviations and Terms

A/P	assessment/plan
Add	additional notes from the doctor or nurse to add to my file
AED	antiepileptic drug
AMA	against medical advice
Asx	asymptomatic
BID	twice a day
BMI	body mass index
c/o	complaints of
CT	or CAT scan, an x-ray scan of your insides
d/c	discontinue
DP	depersonalization, derealization disorder
Dx	diagnosis
ER	emergency room
Etoh	alcohol

F/U	follow up
GAD	generalized anxiety disorder
GP	general practitioner
Hashimotos	an autoimmune disorder where the body attacks the thyroid gland
Hx	history
IC	interstitial cystitis
MD	medical doctor
Mg	milligrams
MRI	magnetic resonance imaging, takes pictures of the insides of your body
MRSA	methicillin-resistant staphylococcus aureus
MVA	motor vehicle accident
N/V	nausea and vomiting
O	"objective," Dr. findings and/or results to tests done in the office
PCP	primary care physician
Po	by mouth
Prn	use when necessary, from the Latin phrase, pro re nata, meaning, "as the circumstance arises"
R/sd	rescheduled
Rr	relative risk
Rx	prescription
S	"subjective," information from the patient's perspective
SA	suicide attempts
SI	suicidal ideation
SS	serotonin syndrome
SSRI	selective serotonin reuptake inhibitor
Synthroid	medicine I take for Hashimotos
UTI	urinary tract infection, misdiagnosis, in my case, of kidney stones

VM	voicemail
W	weight
WHNP	women's health nurse practitioner

List of Doctors

Dr. Aldo, DPT chiropractor.

Dr. Braun, PhD psychologist at the university's counseling center.

Dr. Daus, MD urgent care physician, also Beau's dad.

Dr. Douglas, MD my general practitioner at the university.

Dr. Fiaschetti, MD long-distance, long-term psychiatrist, referred by Dr. Sandy after Dr. Morano has a mental break and nearly kills me with meds, located on the coast, closer to Newport than LA.

Dr. Jane, MD my original general practitioner and the mother of Dr. Scott.

Dr. Jensen, MD psychiatrist who gives me Prozac in tenth-grade, ups the dose and leaves the country.

Dr. Kate, MFT psychologist referred by Dr. Braun, works at BHI on campus (behavioral health institute).

Dr. Morano, MD previous psychiatrist who was tased in his back yard, a general practitioner acting as a psychiatrist.

Dr. Nguyen, MD radiologist.

Dr. Olivera, MD	neurologist.
Dr. Roberts, MD	urgent care physician in Newport.
Dr. Sandy, PhD	beloved psychologist I am linked up with after Portofino rehab stay in high school.
Dr. Scott, MD	long-term general practitioner in Newport, also the son of Dr. Jane, primary care physician who labeled me bipolar after my reaction to Prozac in high school, oversees care while at university.
Dr. Thompson, MD	first psychiatrist I ever visited, in fourth grade because of my sister getting drunk in Palm Springs.
Dr. Whittman, PhD	first psychologist I ever visited, tricked me and sent me to rehab for an eating disorder, reason for my trust issues around therapists.

1 From the Coast to the Hills

...But First, Lexapro...

DR. FIASCHETTI (M.D., PSYCHIATRIST): AUGUST 19, 2009

Lexapro 10mg for anxiety—manic and depressed. (See Appendix A.)
Xanax XR 2-3 mg (See Appendix B.)
No Valium (See Appendix C.)

A Taste Of Fiaschetti's Prescribing Hx

In February, 2009, Dr. Fiaschetti wrote:

> Xanax XR 1mg replaced Valium, which may have worsened IC, preferred Valium but it didn't work the same the second time.

Dr. Fiaschetti did not note when she had prescribed Valium or why. It is referenced in this note after it had been discontinued. But, it is not recorded in my files.

Dr. Fiaschetti liked to skim over details, so this was not a surprise. I also found that this particular doctor, when asked to give a new psychologist, Dr. Braun, my information, completely lied about my background, making me look like someone who needed the medications she prescribed so thoughtlessly. This negligence and outright deceit when informing my new therapist, along with Cathy Fiaschetti's bad attitude when asked for a copy of my records in 2013, made for a less than wholesome impression in retrospect.

Flash forward to the present moment, August 2010, a week before I move from Newport Coast to Los Angeles, Dr. Fiaschetti, my current psychiatrist, starts me on Lexapro.

The Leather Journal: The City of Angels

August 22, 2009

Wow, I am actually moved in.
XO Kali Rae

August 23, 2009

I love it here. I hope I don't get homesick. I love my roommates and I have to and will get a job at MTV or one of the record companies.
XO Kali Rae

Aaron "Shows Me around LA"

Jaxx looks at me with doe eyes, the ones I know so well from our two years together, through thick and thin. He hangs in the doorway, leaning into the room in his dark-colored designer denim and stark white Jack Purcells. "Don't get drunk and forget about me," I hear in my mind. These are the words he said a few days ago in my childhood bedroom in Newport Coast. This time, standing in the doorway of my new apartment, he says nothing before leaving. The heavy door slams shut with a clunk.

I smile. I am moved in!

A notification pops up on my phone from Aaron, the guy who leased me the apartment while wearing Crest Whitestrips. He charmed me into giving him my social media handle so he could message me regarding his offer to show me around LA when I got here and moved in.

My head is pounding. My hair is damp. My ankle is throbbing. I look down to find my foot is purple along the outside edge near my ankle bone running all the way to my pinky toe. I look to the left and Aaron is asleep in his bed.

The night before rushes back without warning but with major holes. There is a gap, blackness, from the time we parked on the steep driveway to his home in the Hills, through the end of the night, with only a few scattered moments in between.

***

Aaron picks me up from my apartment—the same one he leased to me a few weeks prior. He is in a shiny black Audi. He drives straight to his house.

I never imagine anything will go down, not in my wildest nightmares.

I snap back to the present as Aaron wakes up.

"What are you doing?" he asks. He sits up in his bed, looking awful, and looking my way.

"Why am I over here?" I ask.

"You kept hitting me with your foot, so I threw it off the bed. But you kept doing it, so I moved you over there," he says.

"I meant, here, like in your bedroom. What happened last night?" I ask.

"I'm going back to sleep," Aaron says and rolls in his comforter to face the other direction.

***

The sickening feeling in my stomach is growing by the word.

Did this really happen?

I remember Aaron asking me to bring a bathing suit with me, but I didn't think it was a play to get me into bed with him. I remember the Jacuzzi, for a moment, and then nothing: just blackness. (See Appendix H.)

Aaron gives me a strong drink upon arriving. Aaron is not drinking. Situated in the Hollywood Hills, Aaron's home is on the steepest incline I have ever seen. As we park, I wonder how anyone gets in and out of his home without either falling off one end of the property, knocking into the neighbor's mailbox or sliding down the inclined street into the traffic on the busy street below. I wish I would have slid down the driveway and out of this situation, I think, and draw myself into the present moment.

I look back over at Aaron. His fluffy down comforter strikes an odd opposition. It's discordant wrapped around him so cozily. It makes him look harmless, almost angelic. His face is barely visible, and his foot is sticking out at one end. He looks like a very young child, almost a toddler. His blonde curls pushed in front of his eyes. It hurts to see him so vulnerable and to know that when he wakes he will shove all humanness back down to the darkest parts of himself and act like an asshole.

This kind of thing always strikes me. It is the potential that stings; not the potential as a lover, but the potential that this person could be moving the world forward with light. Instead, he is scared. And so, Aaron and others like Aaron spend their lives running away from some wrong someone did to them in their past. Aaron plays the victim and attempts to throw a blanket over the light just like the villain in his past did to him. I snap back into the present moment and toss the small blanket wrapped around my bare waist to the floor.

Stumbling around the messy hardwood floor of his bachelor pad, I gather my jeans and purse. I find them stashed in his closet under his clothes from last night. I sneak out the side door onto the balcony overlooking the hillside. The dew of the morning sticks to me like insulation. All I want to do is wash this away. My head pounds, my vision is shifty, but I rush to get out of there and into my car.

I hold my breath, slowly backing out of the very steep driveway in front of the house. I had no idea this could happen. Worse, it washes over me full-force that Aaron knew exactly what he was doing this entire time. No wonder he refused to hang out with the roommates at my apartment. Aaron's words rush into my mind:

"I'll show you around LA when you move up here," Aaron says motioning for us to head into the next room on the apartment tour. His words are a friendly gesture in a lonely town

No Way Out, Cutting Ties

I can never tell Jaxx what happened.

"Just make sure you don't leave us alone together," I inform Jessica, one of my four roommates. She looks worried. "It's not like Jaxx would hurt me, but depending on his state of mind, he can be a little scary…" I trail off.

"Okay," Jessica says timidly and then builds confidence. "Are you sure this is a good idea?"

"Well, I've refused to see him for a week now. And I need to tell him that it's over in person," I say.

"Yeah, okay. Whatever, Dude. I'm walking down there with you," Jessica says.

Her caution stems from Jaxx's recently intensifying aggression on the phone with me.

Jaxx is planning on moving to LA soon, but at the moment is still living in Orange County. Today, he is visiting me at my apartment.

Jaxx: Downstairs
Me: K one sec

"He's here," I tell Jessica.

"Okay let's go," Jessica says energetically.

I find him outside the side door. He looks more attractive than ever. He's wearing my favorite pair of True Religions, with his Tiffany's dog tag and Jack Purcells.

I immediately regret asking Jessica to be there.

"Hey, Jaxx, how are you?" Jessica chirps.

"Great! And you?" Jaxx says.

"I'm okay, thank you for asking," Jessica responds.

The elevator ride up to our apartment is made more awkward by Jessica's random comments and school-girl gestures.

Once we're inside my apartment, Jaxx and I head to my bedroom. Jessica tags along. Jaxx takes a seat on my bed.

"It's okay," I tell her, so she leaves us alone. After she's gone, I say, "Jaxx, I don't want to be in a relationship when I'm up here, and you're down in Newport. It's too hard, you know? It doesn't make sense."

"Are you kidding?" Jaxx looks down at his clasped hands. "Okay, Kali, whatever you want." Jaxx stands in the doorway for a moment. He shoves his hands into his pockets. I can feel his anger building, "I'm leaving now. Don't be an idiot, Kali. Be safe."

I sit on the bed, in a trance, right where he had been sitting. I hear the door swish and slam shut. The emptiness closes in quickly.

After being taken by men who did not have my permission, I force out the one person who has always been there for me.

What have I done?

Staying with him meant addressing what had gone down while he was away, and I just wasn't willing.

I slam the door on the thoughts before they rush back into my mind.

Jessica walks into my room.

"You okay, girl?" Jessica asks.

"Yeah, I think… Not really, actually, but things are changing. I'll be okay," I say.

Clinging to Home

"What are you doing?" Dane asks.

Dane Edwards is the mid-twenties guy who lives directly across the hall from me and my roommates, with his dog, Harley.

Silence.

"Come back to bed, It's like five a.m.," he half whispers. I'm unsure if his tone is due to the time of morning or the caution with which he is handling the situation.

I say nothing.

I'm lying face up on someone's living room floor, da Vinci pose, feet angled toward his bedroom just slightly. I make no effort to acknowledge him but can see out of my periphery that he's wearing white boxer briefs, standing in his doorway, not a step farther, just close enough for me to catch a vague idea of what he is wearing.

"You're so weird." Dane sighs and walks back into his room.

"I can't get into my apartment," I say to myself.

I don't have the energy to repeat it loud enough for him to hear. Nor do I care if he hears. I feel nothing, absolutely nothing. Well, I feel a slight headache, soon to be an intense headache, I didn't sleep last night. Well, I hadn't been conscious enough to sleep. The whole thing feels like one big swirling, nauseating nightmare. I dare to dive into the darkroom of my mind to develop the night before.

I remember pieces. But more so, I remember feeling as if my soul left my body, utter lifelessness. And the color, I remember the color of last night: pure black, no light reflecting from another room, no nightlight, no cell phone screen, just black.

The majority of the night I am too disoriented to decipher whether I am lying horizontal, vertical, or sideways on the bed, with my head where my feet should be. The times I find which direction I am facing, I nearly vomit. The Earth is way too steady for me to handle. I am floating away somewhere. I lie motionless as my body tries to find itself in space. I am not awake, surely not asleep, but I cannot find gravity.

I snap back into the present.

My subconscious scolds me.

Get up and get water like a reasonable person. Then, go home.

Nope. Not going to happen. I have no physical energy, and I am drained mentally. There is no way I will be able to talk my body into moving. Not now.

About five minutes pass. Louder this time: "I can't get into my apartment. I'll knock again in a few minutes." My voice trails off for the second part. Who was I talking to anyway? Dane certainly didn't care.

"Sleeping. Come sleep or don't," Dane says from his room.

A few minutes later I muster enough energy to get to my feet. Whoa: I feel awful. I stand in the same spot for about a minute, steadying myself against his marble bar. The empty eight-ounce glasses are still there, just about a centimeter of brownish-amber liquid remain in the bottom. The smell is overwhelmingly putrid. I almost lose it.

I open his heavy door and slip around it, closing it as carefully as possible but waiting for its inevitable slam.

Clunk. Click.

Why do these doors have to shut themselves so loudly?!

I walk a few steps forward and knock.

"God, please, why can't somebody just let me in…" I moan and turn around to return to Dane's awful-smelling apartment.

"Kali! Oh my god!" Jessica shouts.

I turn back around to find Jessica in our doorway. Her pink plaid pajama bottoms and band shirt look extra comfortable in this particular moment.

"Thank God. Thank you, Jessica. I feel awful," I mumble. My eyes meet hers for only a quick instant before casting down onto the ground again. I can't handle myself anymore.

"What. The. Fuck. Girl. What happened to you last night?! We were so worried about you! And wait, Dane?! What? Is that good? Oh my god. Like, was—" Jessica begins to work herself into a frenzy that I can't handle at the moment.

"I don't want to talk about it. I need sleep," I say. I trudge forward into my apartment, "I think I'm going to be sick."

I dodge her, sprinting through my shared room with Stephanie and into the master bathroom and puking whiskey and bile into the brand new toilet.

"Kali?" I hear Stephanie whisper.

I am so jealous of Stephanie and her grogginess I can't even stand it.

"AAAAUUUUHHGG!" I muster.

Coming out of the bathroom in the master bedroom of my apartment, I hear Stephanie snoring again. I head over to my bed on the opposite side of the room. My furniture is only half set up. I have a bedside table, a new desk, office chair, and bed. I look at the setup, feeling disgust as I remember how helpful my father had been in helping me buy and set up my new room. My heart sinks, and I push every emotion away, overwhelmed, before heading to fetch the medication in the drawer built into my Ikea bedframe.

There is no way this many awful things have already happened. Isn't there a reset button on this whole life thing?

The sound of empty plastic bottles hitting up against one another is extra loud as I pull the drawer open. The sound deepens the pain in my gut. I unzip the makeup bag containing my Rite Aid medication bottles. Now more than ever, I need to take something. I go through the medication bottles one at a time: Xanax? Empty. Ativan? Empty. Valium? Empty. There is not even a little bit of a crushed Xanax left. Nothing. Zilch. Nada.

I hate LA.

I want to erase the past month, wash out my insides leave them in the sunshine to dry. Get me out of here.

Dane Edwards: The Dick across the Hall

I wake up to a text message later that same day.
Dane: I can't believe you didn't suck my dick last night. Really, Life?

I can't even react, other than to think that's randomly awful. Jogging my memory takes a bit of energy, but I don't remember past sitting on his couch, drinking whiskey sours and watching *Royal Pains* episodes. Then I remember what he is referring to. The night before, too drunk to refuse anything, I had refused to perform fellatio on him.

"No, I don't do that. I refuse to do that," I say, sure of myself. I reply quickly, in hopes that the speed of my answer voids his initial embarrassing question and forces it to retreat into his supposedly mature and caring mouth.
It shakes me. But not enough. Dane smiles a megawatt smile and chuckles, easing my anxiety about the interaction with my new neighbor. "I'm just playing!" Dane says, laughs a little more and refills my whiskey drink, the special one he made for us while binge-watching a show on his wide screen with his boxer, Harley.

The couch smells like brand new leather. Dane's cologne is musky but sweet. His apartment, just across the hall from mine, is my safety zone within this new city. Especially after the Aaron night. The night when Aaron posed as my friend to show me around the city, and instead, treated me like a disposable camera after having sex with my unconscious body, and then apparently, throwing my ankle so hard off his bed that the encounter lefts a fist-sized bruise and an inch-long cut to boot.

That can never happen again.

I should have known.

You should have known, my mind echoes. No, it's fine, I assure myself. I'm sure Aaron is a kind man who simply made a mistake.

I remember staring at my phone a few seconds longer when I texted Aaron to ask if he would hang at my apartment with my roommates and me instead of my going to his place.

Aaron: Let's go to my place. Bring a bathing suit. :)

No, I reassure myself after my mind questions his planned out approach. He had at least planned to get me in a bathing suit. It's okay; he is probably in love with me. Aaron probably can't figure out why he can't stop thinking about me, which is why—wait—he hasn't called or texted me back since that night. It's okay, Aaron just had no idea that I am not that type of girl, that's all.

I should not have gone to his apartment alone, and although I barely remember even putting on a bathing suit, I should not have been in that situation. I should have known. But Aaron will call me and make it all feel better. My mind battles itself attempting to put together the emotional pieces that seem to be ruining my days in the new city.

I snap back into the moment and the text from Dane on my cellphone screen. I look down at the text again. My blood runs cold one more time. I don't flinch before swiftly deleting the conversation, hoping it will delete the night before along with it. I made it clear to Dane before last night that I didn't want to do anything with him. The boundary-setting conversation took place only a few days ago. Obviously, nothing has changed.

The Leather Journal: Initiation into the City

August 27, 2009

Well I've moved in. I went back to Newport today ... and for some reason I'm really sad.

I had sex with Aaron the first night I was with him and even though he is super nice and isn't bailing on me, I wish I hadn't done that. But I'm trying not to have any regrets.

Being single is difficult, especially after I broke up with my opiate dealer who spent the first few nights here.

Okay, so I slept at Aaron's two nights in a row and then a day later, last night, I got drunk again and slept at Dane's [the next door neighbor.] We didn't have sex. I like him a lot. I told him no. But I wish I had been able do the same with Aaron.

I really, really wish I wasn't all out of Xanax, Valium and Ativan. I didn't sleep at all last night at Dane's and I can't sleep now at all either.

And, finally, I feel a little bad about my situation with Jaxx. I did love him at a point in my life, but it totally burned out and became a very unhealthy relationship. I only wanted him for his drugs or because I was selfish and lonely.

I really just wish I could do things that I approve of once in a while, just so that I could get out of my own head, and not be depressed. I keep remembering Jaxx telling me not to get drunk in LA and forget about him and that's exactly what I did.

I'm not okay.

I never said anything back to him, and that is how it turned out.

How did any of this happen?

I hate relationships.

I hate LA.

Later:

So, it's around eight o'clock and Dane can't hang out because he says he is working until midnight and his roommate's mom is spending the night.

Jaxx called but I had to be strong and not pick it up or call back.

Aaron, who I very much regret now ... very much regret, called all hammered and called me Ashley and then said that Ashley was just his cousin who had texted him at the same time I called.

I am just super scared I have an STD from Aaron. But I need to stay calm because I know that I don't and I'm freaking out for no reason and that he will call me later and tomorrow and he's not a liar and he will apologize.

Dane isn't lying either; he is working late.

XO Kali Rae
(See Appendices A, B, C, D.)

August 31, 2009

I can't write.
XO Kali Rae
(See Appendix A.)

EMERGENCY ROOM: SEPTEMBER 7, 2009
Emergency Room Visit
Dx: Pyelonephritis (kidney infection) (See Appendix E.)
Rx: Cipro (See Appendix M.)

DR. FIASCHETTI: SEPTEMBER 16, 2009
Seroquel 50 mg at bedtime and 25 mg during the day. (See Appendix F.)

Overprescribing Seriously Dangerous Medications

The prescription for Lexapro, resulting in a completely unhinged version of myself, followed immediately by a prescription for a powerful antipsychotic, really sets the tone right for Dr. Fiaschetti. She should have tapered me off Lexapro, the heavy SSRI that has now been linked to an incredibly high number of serotonin syndrome cases as well as the false diagnosis of bipolar disorder in depressed adolescents who were given the drug for depression (See Appendix A.) Lexapro is also linked to an increase in suicidal ideation and an increase in actual suicides. And those are just the two most appalling side effects from a superficial point of view.

Seroquel comes with its own massive number of adverse reactions, false marketing campaigns, FDA fines and billion-dollar lawsuits. Instead of checking anything other than the encyclopedia full of medications on her bookshelf, Dr. Fiaschetti prescribes Seroquel, to take during the day, because I am manic. (See Appendix F.)

Taking Care of My Health, a Personal Trainer

I flinch and glance to the right instinctively. It is a conditioned reaction, to look up at your perpetrator, one that gets thwarted when you realize the person isn't going to stop, even if you threaten him with that evil glance thrown his way. I bite my tongue and inhale.

I look pale in the mirror of the cold gym this morning. It frightens me, but I look back down to my knuckles turning white. I'm in a straight-armed plank position stretching my calves. It is five a.m. on a Tuesday, and I am feeling the side effects of an all-nighter fueled by Adderall and coffee.

"Well looks like you're going to need to run some of this off," Jason says.

Jason is pushing down hard with one hand on the small of my back, his fingers shifting way too close to the wrong places.

"I can't run. I told you already," I say.

"Don't pull that with me. I'm training you. Remember that," Jason says. Jason fastens his grip fast around my left hip. His hands are so big that he holds me up with one hand. His fingers dig into my hip joint aggressively.

"I just had knee surgery," I say.

"We will jog then. Up you go," Jason says. He pulls me up, almost throwing me into the mirrored walls of his apartment's gym-room. "Turn around. One more thing…"

I naively do as I am told, exhausted and wanting to please him, for a reason, God only knows.

He has a whiteboard in his apartment. It is divided into seven vertical sections. In each column, there are lists of names with times and school-related things scribbled in. Underneath is his personal workout for the day.

His apartment is always impeccably clean.

I long for the structure of his life. It is all so simple and planned out. Nothing less and nothing more than what is written on the whiteboard gets accomplished each day. But he sure as hell accomplishes each one of the things written down.

If I come over on a Wednesday, there are blue lines through each of the names and homework assignments, as well as things like "Leg Day."

I admire his work ethic and his ability to stay motivated while busy working at his career, living alone, and studying in college. I also enjoy messing up his plans. I like begging him to relax about having his perfectly proportioned dinner consumed by five p.m. at the latest.

Jason is comedy to me, because I feel in my soul that nothing, especially not life, can be controlled in the precise way he is attempting. Jason doesn't have parents, he says, and he comes from Boston.

To me, Jason is a big, muscly, orphan, and I eat his story all up.

He cranes his head to the left and then straight up, raising his eyebrows real quick, before shaking it off and reciting, like an actor would, in a way too stereotypical scene, in a Lifetime movie (if they did fitness films).

"Okay, let's go! What are you waiting for?" Jason says.

I stand up and cross my arms over my chest, covering my chest instinctively. "I'm not running today," I say.

"Then why are you here? Why are you paying me to train you if you won't follow what I'm telling you to do?" Jason asks.

"I have an injury that has gotten a lot worse since working with you; my chiropractor told me not to run. I don't know how to answer your questions…" I say.

…maybe because I feel bad for you. I say the last part in my head as I glance to the ground next to his washed and rewashed, knock-off Nikes. It makes my heart ache.

"Well then, why don't you plan your session today," Jason says. "How bout we do things your way?"

"Jason! I just can't run! I can do legs, arms, abs…anything, you name it! I'll do it! Just not running!" I shout.

"Get on the ground. Lie on your back," Jason says.

I slowly get back onto the black rubber gym floor, rolling my eyes in the process. "You know this isn't life or death—" I say.

"We are going to do something new," Jason says.

He gets down on one knee, like a wrestling coach. "But first..." He grabs my right foot and quickly swoops it off the mat and up toward my shoulder. "We stretch," he says.

Forcing a Milkshake; Control Freak Clues

At six a.m. I finish up my early morning workout with Jason Murray. Workouts with Jason are a new start for me. My plan is to transform my health and to get my head back on straight. It has been a tough couple of months.

I am exhausted. The session turned intense, even without running, very intense. I am ready to get home and sleep for an hour before school.

I know this will be the last time I will ever come back to Jason as a trainer. He has pushed me over the top somehow, a nearly impossible feat; since I am known to push myself, physically, harder than anyone I know. There is something more than the exercise; something else is bothering me.

Every time I step into the gym with him I feel uncomfortable in my skin. And I finally began to identify the guilty feeling in my stomach when I saw myself in the mirrored room this morning.

The darkness of the early morning doesn't help. I felt exposed from the moment I saw Jason Murray. I felt ashamed. It used to be different. He used to be kind. Right?

I had no idea that Jason had acquired a brewing hatred for me. What did I do?

Jason grabs my biceps and furrows his brow.

"You look too thin. You need to be eating two thousand more calories a day than you are," he says. Soliciting a response that I am not selling. He jerks my arm to get me to look at him and continues, "Starting today."

He grabs my forearm swiftly again, painfully this time and like he's reprimanding a child for stealing a cookie out of the cookie jar.

"Okay, no, I just gained five pounds. I've never actually been heavier, but whatever, sure," I retort.

I don't care and will try to eat more, but I hadn't asked him to comment on my figure. The idea that he did, makes me angrier by the moment. I swing my arm viciously out of his grasp.

"Let go, Jason!" I shout.

"Geez. You PMSing?" Jason says.

I instantly feel I've overreacted, "No. Sorry. I don't like when people grab me," I say.

I recently gained weight. I am looking better than ever. I don't mention it because it would seem arrogant.

"Anyway, you may have gained weight Kali, but you need to put on at least ten more pounds to be, well..." looking me up and down, "in a good place—" Jason says.

"Okay...cool. Will do. Thanks again!" I say as I exit.

Asshole.

I pick up my gym bag, hand him my mother's check and step out of the muggy private gym into the cool, blue morning.

"Why don't you come back to my apartment?" he says. Seeing that I'm not too excited, he adds, "I need to see that you'll do it." He lowers his tone, still waiting for me to turn around. "I'll make you a protein shake with extra calories. I mean chocolate. I'll make you a chocolate shake, my treat," he says.

I'm still not buying it.

"Don't worry. They're good calories. You worked out hard today. Come on!" He sounds friendly again, even playful, like a puppy. I feel bad disowning him. I want him to feel he's helping me. Would a free dairy-free, gluten-free, soy-free milkshake hurt anyone?

I turn back around to face him having almost made it past the doorframe. I step back inside.

"Okay, I guess that's fine," I say.

It is a kind gesture to be worried about my caloric intake.

"Come back inside then. Help me clean up," Jason says.

He holds out three five-pound weights like they're marbles.

"Put these on that stack," he says.

"UGH!"

We walk back to his apartment as the sun just begins to reveal itself through the dark early morning fog. I feel like a puppy on a short leash. It's refreshing to be controlled by somebody like this. He is my personal trainer. It's not like he's trying to control me as a person.

Yeah, no problems here. Jason just wants to do his job right, I assure myself. And I am technically his responsibility right now…fitness-wise.

He watches me intensely as I gulp down the disgusting drink he blended for me. Hands on his hips, he demands I drink every last drop. I hold the slim glass up to my eyes and watch the thick mixture accumulate in a sludge pool at the bottom of the glass.

Peering into the 1/8 inch of liquid left, "Really, Jason?" I say.

This last part is like climbing Mount Everest sick from HAPE and HACE (inside joke). There is a raw egg in the mixture, and I feel it immediately. I hold my nose to finish.

"Good. Grab your things. I need to go. Eat six hundred more calories than usual today," Jason says.

"Yeah, okay," I say. The door to his ground-floor apartment slams shut behind us. "Damn that's a heavy door."

An Alarming Phone Call

Regardless of the few weird sessions with Jason as a trainer, I am so desperate to get out of my apartment that I start studying at his apartment after class. His apartment makes for a nice getaway from the roommates. Since we are in a few of the same classes and partnered in the environmental club, it makes sense. This way, if we have to study late, I can sleep on the couch to wake up for my now five a.m. training sessions. I trust Jason implicitly. He is organized, mature and my personal trainer.

It is a phone call that I receive while back home in Newport Coast that shakes up the haven up a bit.

"Hey!" I answer the phone.

"Hey! I've got to tell you something," Jason says.

"Okay. Shoot," I say.

"I bought a gun," Jason says.

"What! Why?!" I almost shout into the phone.

"I talked with my friend, and he explained how much better it is for me to be protected..." Jason says.

"No, why?" I ask again.

He laughs. "And I learned how to use it," he says.

"Okay, Jason. You don't need a gun. What are you talking about?" I say.

He's laughing harder now, "Kali, Kali! I got a gun!"

"Stop. Return the gun. Why do you need a gun? That's illegal. Isn't that illegal?" I say.

Click.

What the fuck just happened?

I rush to rationalize why he called. He is from Boston. He lives alone. He got mugged once. I start putting the pieces of my logical puzzle together. I am somehow able to create a reason for the call, to rationalize the conversation.

I will see him in two days for training anyway. I'll get him to return it. Weird. Super weird, though.

Two days after the odd phone call with Jason, I am back in LA at Jason's apartment working.

I want you to go down on me," Jason says, out of the blue, as I am hunched over my English essay.

"What? No. I don't do that," I say.

"Do it for me," Jason says.

"No. Stop. Do it yourself," I say.

He laughs indignantly and starts rummaging in the top drawer of his desk across the room from me. I am on the carpet, legs sprawled, the usual writing pose, killing two birds with one stone: stretching and homework. But after his comment, I scoot my legs together, uncomfortable.

Time slows to a stop. Jason is walking toward me, holding a black handgun and smiling overzealously.

"Is that real? Jason, what are you doing?" I ask. My heart beats hard, but I slow it down to regulate him. He does not respond. My heart begins thumping quicker. "Jason, please put that down."

He stands over me, the gun hanging by his side in his right hand, muscles bulging from his obsessive workouts and raw egg mixtures. He grabs me by the shoulder and tosses me onto the bed.

I let out a sound I've never made before, more of a stifled pleading than anything. I am perched up on my elbow. He doesn't set the gun down as he unzips his pants.

"Do it," Jason says. He brings the gun right up to the place between my eyebrows. The gun is cold.

"Please stop," I say. Jason doesn't move the gun, "Jason, please put that down. You don't want to do this. Trust me."

"You know what this is called?" Jason asks.

"No," I respond.

"It's called a Glock. I got special bullets for it," Jason says.

"Jason, please stop. This is getting really bad," I say.

I move my chest toward him to try and scoot out from underneath him, but he jams his other hand into my chest, and I crumple to the bed.

"You don't want to do this," I say again before I leave my body.

I go numb. I am unfeeling now. I accept what might happen. I inhale deeply and pray silently;

I love you; I love you, Jesus Christ, please come into my heart, I love you… I love you.

I silently recite a jumble of prayers as Jason continues rambling on about something. He's torn my clothes off now, but I haven't felt a thing. He reaches the arm without the gun under my torso, flipping me over in one motion.

"Get on your knees, ass up!" he demands.

I follow his directions and yell as he jams himself into me. I feel the gun brushing against my neck.

I am unafraid, unfeeling…planning.

He is so much bigger than me, six foot three and probably two hundred and ten pounds, all muscle; there is no way I will be able to hurt him enough to get out from under his grasp. I am okay with being shot if I am shot as I am leaving; that doesn't worry me.

Jason finishes and lets out a strange sound. Having flipped back over, I see his hand is still holding the gun, but he has it resting on the bed as he recovers. The pressure on it makes me nervous; the mattress is deeply indented with the weight of the weapon.

This is my time.

I hoist myself up. But before I can move off the bed, he jams the gun into my forehead again.

"Stop!" Jason shouts. I watch his finger press down on the trigger.

I slam my eyes shut without enough time to wince. An image of my mother, father, sister and brother together at the dinner table at our house on Seacrest Lane displays itself like a painting in my mind as I wait.

And I hear it.

Click.

Exhale.

Things go black.

I jolt my eyes open. Jason is holding the gun up to my forehead still, but now he's moving it onto its side. He's staring at it, intensely, angrier than I've ever seen him.

Unexpected Game of Russian Roulette

"I bought bullets. They are right here," Jason says. He retreats from the bed and walks over to the drawer where he had retrieved the gun. Sure enough, he pulls out a carton that I can only compare with the staple gun refills in my top drawer.

I don't dare to move as he is only feet away and I am not big enough to fight him off.

To my surprise, Jason looks at me and laughs. He throws me an old basketball t-shirt. For some reason, the gesture seems extra caring. I thank him, throwing it over my head as I sit up, legs crossed and knees clenching tightly together. I wrap my arms around my shins.

He is pacing back and forth in front of the drawer. Out of nowhere, he carefully places the gun back into the drawer and walks over to the kitchen. It is a studio apartment, so the kitchen is just a little offset to the left.

Like nothing has happened, Jason starts making his protein shake. I am shaking like a leaf as he peels the banana and scoops his chocolate powder into the blender, turning it on calmly. His demeanor is completely different.

"You want a shake?" he asks.

"No, I'm okay," I say.

He sips the shake while staring at me out of the corner of his eye. He seems to be sizing up my emotional state. His eyes have softened immensely, and he seems worried about me. And then, like a light switch, he slams his empty plastic cup down onto the bar.

"You are wearing my shirt, and you are sitting on my bed." He's mad again, sort of.

"I can take it off. I just thought you wanted me to…" I say.

"And you are in my space," Jason continues.

"I don't…I can leave. I'll go right now," I respond.

"Don't leave! Stay here. Stay right there," Jason orders.

He approaches the bed and turns around, walking toward the same drawer. My stomach clenches and I feel a wash of missed opportunity. He collapses into the desk chair pulled out from his desk, jutting his elbows into his thighs; palms pressed firmly together, thumbs set on his third eye. Looking at the ground, he pushes himself up and walks back toward me on the bed. After rummaging through the left bedside drawer, Jason picks up a Bible. Still avoiding looking my direction, he sits down at the top of the bed and opens up the burgundy, hardbound book.

I glance around the room. I have a clear path to the door. If the door is unlocked, I can run. My eyes dart down to my large book bag and purse, with years of practice sweeping them up to run to the next class on time, I know I could grab them on the way out, no problem.

I am shocked out of planning as Jason begins to repeat a passage to himself, nod, and read it again.

"Hmmm," he says, "hmmm," flipping back the page to read it again.

Okay, I've got one shot.

Adrenaline pulses through my veins.

On the count of three. One…Two…Fuck it.

I simultaneously bound off of the bed and swoop up my bags.

Shit!

The front door won't open.

It's locked!! The handle is stuck!

I fumble with the lock embedded in the handle.

It's stuck!

I jam it up and down and pushing with all of my might, jamming my right shoulder into the door. My hands are shaking, but I manage to turn the silver deadbolt to the right and then left. In a stroke of luck, the door swings open. My bag catches the door, and it slams onto my left index finger. I yelp and yank it out of the door frame. There's blood, but I don't care.

I sprint down the gray-carpeted hallways, past the broken fountain outside of the gym. I finally get to the lock on the metal gates to the street where I parallel-parked that morning.

The early morning sun is far from rising.

I fumble to put my car in drive, shaking from head to toe. My finger is pulsing.

I don't feel the pain until I am far out of range of the apartment parking lot.

I look at my hands, and my left index finger is cracked up to the cuticle. My first knuckle is swollen and burgundy. Blood is dripping onto the steering wheel.

I sob all the way to my apartment.

When I get to my apartment, I wipe the blood off of the steering wheel and center console. The only injury I sustained is my pointer finger, which is now throbbing in pain. I break down in the parking structure, overwhelmed that I'm alive and so grateful, for once, to be within the walls of that cement structure.

I fall asleep in the parking garage of my Santa Monica apartment draped in Jason's oversized men's basketball jersey.

Stacked Lesions

A couple of weeks later, the chiropractor finds me out. I deny everything as he points out the "traumatic"† stacked lesions in my cervical and lumbar spine. I am also diagnosed with a neck sprain and have to have my coccyx painfully repositioned.

Stacked lesions (or allopathic legions) are places in the spine where there is significant misalignment resulting from compounding injuries sustained to multiple vertebrate in one section of the spine. In my case, the multiple stacked lesions refer to areas of injury in my cervical, lumbar and sacral spine.

"You can talk to me, Kali," he says.

I stare at my toes from the lying-down position. The doctor helps me up and continues, "Kali, you couldn't have done these things to yourself. And the bruises you have are troubling to me…"

"I bruise super easily," I say.

"Not like this, you don't. I need to see you looking better the next time I see you or I'm going to have to get someone involved. And trust me, I don't want to have to do that," the doctor says.

Knock. Knock.

---

† as in medically traumatic or trauma-induced

"Everything okay, Doc?" my mom asks, appearing in the doorway.

It took four years for that finger to heal. When it did, the fingernail grew this funny, wave-like bump over the older nail: a constant reminder. This part eventually grew all the way out, too. It was only last year that the last part of the deformed nail grew long enough to cut off.

Bodies heal so much more easily than our minds.

AYN ALDO (CHIROPRACTOR, M.S. D.P.T.): NOVEMBER 2009

Note: dancer, h/o [history of] knee surgery, hip pain, neck sprain
Diagnosis: multiple stacked lesions and bruises on skin, patient counseled r/g injuries sustained.
Plan: 3xs week, therapy and exercises, rest

The Leather Journal: Neglected

November 15, 2009

It's been a while, I apologize.
XO Kali Rae

Missing Jaxx, Jay Gatsby

Lying on my back in my cousin's vacant bedroom, I stare up at the ceiling.

Could this happen? Jaxx and I, again?

I pick up the medicine ball, thanks to the multiple stacked lesions from Jason and the ensuing physical therapy visits with Ayn Aldo. I'm supposed to use the ball nightly. I roll it under my shoulder blades.

Jaxx moved up to LA about a month ago. I overheard this when I met with a mutual friend of ours, Alexa, Jaxx's new roommate. I did not know they were living together when I went to see Alexa one night, lonely as ever and wanting to touch base with someone from the same town who is now in the big city.

Jaxx and I have not seen each or spoken to each other since the day I broke up with him in August.

The last few months have felt like it had been an eternity. Every time I think of Jaxx, I go back to a place where, although I am a mess, the people around me are safe. When Jaxx was there, I was safe. Since Jaxx's departure, the very last pieces of myself have been taken by strangers.

The padding that lined the little room in my insane asylum had turned into sticky spikes. People see me as a target, as a desperate person they can profit from; they don't know me. They don't recognize my family name; they don't comprehend my background. They don't care to help me find my way.

My new "friends" mock me and use me like a circus animal. They put me on display, instead of holding out their hand. I am sinking in quicksand, and they are calling people over to watch. The whole time, I just wanted somebody to hold on to; I wanted to find home again.

Los Angeles is not Newport Coast.

Back in His Atmosphere

As I shut the red door to my aunt's house, I'm surprised by the matte black Mercedes S-Class with its silver rims and blacked-out windows. It's stealthy but romantic in the dusk of that magical autumn night in Mar Vista. I hesitate to walk over to it since I can't see inside. The driver's window rolls down and Jaxx puts up his hand, a signal that it's him.

He opens the heavy door and gets out to hold it for me. I get in and am immediately hit with a rush of scents: leather, new car, my favorite cologne, and tobacco, faintly.

He looks perfect, his hair straightened and newly cut. His smile overwhelms me.

"How have you been?" Jaxx asks.

I have to collect myself and cross my legs before responding. "Good! Wow, nice car!" I say.

"Yeah, thanks. So do you want to go to Teddy's? I've been working as a promoter up here with Stephen. You wanna finally check it out?" Jaxx asks.

"Sure! Where is it?" I ask.

"Hollywood and Vine. Let's do it," Jaxx says.

"I'm not dressed to go out at all," I laugh, looking down at my comfy, over-sized sweater, denim shorts.

"You look perfect, always Kali. Anyway, you look famous. We can just pretend you're famous," Jaxx reassures me.

I then see my awkward boot-sandals. I immediately regret that decision.

Damn, Jaxx is always so composed. He is so cool that it makes me feel fashionable. Jaxx is a mix between Edward Cullen and Nick Gatsby but raised in Southern California, much more mellow, and he is mine.

The City Of Stars

Halfway through the journey into Hollywood from the Westside, Jaxx offers me something to help with my headache. As I pop the pill into my mouth and chew. The sour, grainy, smooth paste gets stuck in my molars. I swish water around my mouth to get the flavor to die down. It is an awful taste, but the feelings associated with it are so good that I don't mind.

I enjoy it. It takes me back to a time where things felt warm and safe, where none of those men could have ever gotten near me.

The sun shines until the last moment it's swallowed by the night. I'm grateful I brought my gold aviators.

The effect one of those pills is like this: You clip in (take pill), wait, maybe slightly inching forward on the tracks, the part of the roller coaster before it stars moving (wait) and then…

BAM!

You accelerate from zero mph to the top speed, before your stomach can catch up. Except with opiates, instead of moving quickly all at once, you slow down all at once. The opiate hits you and all the pain of the day washes away, along with your inhibitions. Simultaneously, your love receptors, dopamine, skyrocket.

I melt into Jaxx's Rolex as he powerfully works the stick shift. He is in charge again. I will marry him on the spot if he asks. I am just happy to be home again.

The Red Cap

"The toilet is broken! What are you doing in there?" I ask.

"I'm going to the bathroom! I'll be out in a minute!" Jaxx says.

I feel a familiar sensation in the pit of my stomach. "Jaxx! Come out of the bathroom. Please!" I yell.

He opens the door looking hazy.

"What's up, baby?" Jaxx says.

A red cap falls to the carpet from his hipster lapel pocket, and he stumbles to pick it up quickly, stuffing it into his back pocket.

"Jaxx what is that?" My voice is shaking, "What is that, Jaxx. Tell me right now!"

"Relax...relax, babe. It's just a paper clip," Jaxx says.

"A fucking paper clip? Really, Jaxx?" I say.

I reach around him to get to his back pocket. He holds my hands.

"Kali, relax. It's nothing," Jaxx says. His sticks his hands into both his pockets and pulls them out. "Look." He flashes his palms and then flips his hands over several times, "See, nothing."

"It isn't in that pocket! It fell out of the one on your shirt!" I shout.

"Kali, nothing's there," Jaxx says. He reaches into his shirt pocket. "Look. You can check me, nothing's there. You're seeing things, babe."

"You moved it! I saw you!" I say.

I reach around him into his pockets, as he holds his hands up, slightly mocking me. I find nothing.

His pockets are empty except for a couple receipts and crumpled up cash. But he looks terrible and I know better. He was in the bathroom for twenty minutes. The toilet is broken. Mostly, I just know better. I have gone through this before and I know this isn't a sober Jaxx.

He moves toward me arms, open for an embrace. His eyes terrify and disgust me at the same time. I pity him but I hate him for lying and I want so badly for this all to not be what it obviously has become.

"No!" I rush out of the hallway. "I'm not doing this again. How could you?" I say.

"Kali, baby, what are you talking about?" Jaxx says. He is too calm for what has just occurred.

"Let's go to Urth Cafe. Babe. Babe. Stop. Please stop, don't do this," Jaxx begs. I turn around and he is standing there looking so thirsty for affection. "Kali, Kali, Kali. Come here."

I reluctantly fall into his comfortable embrace. He thinks he's won and maybe he has. I am completely and utterly devastated, AGAIN. And this time, by the person who broke me in the first place. I crumple my shoulders into his chest.

"Baby, let's go shopping. I want to buy you something," he says.

I say nothing.

My head buried in his chest, all I can see are his glazed-over eyes. It is the worst thing I have seen since the last time I saw that look in his eyes. He is killing himself and unknowingly taking me along with him.

Trials with Gatsby

I let the door slam behind me as I walk, defeated, out of his apartment. How could you have let this happen again?

At my car I swing my load of books into the back seat of my old Range Rover.

Where is my medicine?

I frantically shovel through my oversized bag, throwing notes and lip balm , journals, and perfume samples onto the floorboards.

I need my medicine.

I NEED MY MEDICINE.

I am beginning to whimper in frustration and defeat. My fingers stumble into the little, round pill case.

Gotcha!

For an instant, I feel better. I shove two small blue pills into my mouth. I can't swallow, dry mouth, and there is no water around anywhere. I gulp continuously, but to no avail.

I end up in tears, sobbing and chewing up the Xanax in the same breath. In a lowly parking lot, on the sketchy side of Olympic Blvd. in West Los Angeles. He isn't chasing after me. The door to the parking garage isn't swinging open.

Even if he is coming to find me, it won't be the real Jaxx. He will look childish: red eyes, messy hair, bad posture. That Jaxx is repulsive to me. But

I have seen the other side, and it is so desirable, so polished, that I can't get myself to drive away from him.

I sit folded over the steering wheel in Jaxx's apartment parking lot for more than a few minutes before deciding it will look better to drive somewhere else to have a complete meltdown, a meltdown fueled by my now ex-boyfriend's drug cabinet and my psychiatrist's lazy attempt to fit me into a category.

I make it halfway down the street before tears cloud my vision enough that I am forced me to pull over.

I sob and eat another blue pill, sob, then take an orange one. I need to stay awake.

I stare at my phone as if I'm searching to find myself or God, or both. I desire with every ounce of myself for something to appear that I will not accept anyway.

The trust between Jaxx and me is shattered for the second time, and we all know the saying.

I quickly regret the orange pill and rifle through the glove compartment to find the bottle of opiates Jaxx allotted me for the week we would be apart.

Jaxx has moved to LA, but he has been very busy working with his cousin, or so he said.

I take a couple pain pills from the bottle, chew them and force myself to taste the bitter chunks of grainy powder. It becomes caulk in my mouth as I wait for the pain to subside like usual.

Thirty minutes pass while I'm stopped on a random street. I test the radio out. A hit country music song wails through the speakers. I break down into puddles of gut-busting sobs once more.

Why aren't the pills working?!

I mute the radio.

Usually, by this point, I feel or at least start feeling thoroughly loved—like a baby swaddled in a blanket. Tonight it feels as if I am all wrapped up in that blanket, but no one is around. The feeling that comes with being wrapped in a warm blanket is not here at all. I feel deserted. The drugs are not working.

HOW THE FUCK DO I DO THIS?

I cannot stop the flood of memories as my mind runs through the file cabinet of the past two years. I find that I've filed away a majority of the moments Jaxx and I spent together, already, knowing full-well that I would never be able to bring them back. Not the way they were. The awareness of this causes the pain to intensify.

Twenty minutes later, a familiar Mercedes Benz pulls up next to mine.

"Come on. Get in. We'll pick your car up later," Jaxx says.

The Night Is Young

He looks a lot better than he did. His eyes are clearer. His voice has energy and a responsible vibe about it. I feel as if he can truly take care of me, protect me. I stumble out of my car and into his.

Whoa, I am wobbly.

"You good?" he asks protectively, having gotten out of his car to open the door for me.

"Yeah, I'm good," I say. I slur my way back into his car and back into his life, at least for the night.

Hours later I am doubled over, in the same parking lot I had zoomed out of earlier in the evening, throwing up my guts onto the pavement. I took too many pills.

Coming to from a blackout, I can't see anyone around, but Jaxx's car is speeding out of the parking structure.

Did we fight?

A few moments later, clunk, clunk. His car reappears in the garage. He parks and looks angry, rushing over to me.

"You're actually fucking sick? This is incredible," Jaxx says.

I look up at Jaxx and the world turns in on itself. I open and close my eyes, hoping the feeling will pass.

I recognize the bright lights illuminating the familiar grocery store.

I know where this is!

"Hey!" I straighten up out of my slouch onto the passenger-side door. "Why are we at my apartment?" "I am dropping you off," Jaxx says.

"At fucking Ralph's?" I ask.

"You can walk through. Get yourself some water before you go home," he says.

This is true, but I am mad at him. Why is he deserting me? a

I glance at the clock.

At 10:45 at night? What happened?

I quite literally fall out of the car and realize he has driven me in my Range Rover to the back of my apartment building: to Ralph's.

I guess I don't have to worry about picking up my car up.

"Wait, No! What are you doing?!" I shout.

"You need sleep, call me when you wake up," Jaxx says coldly and holds my keys out in front of my face dangling them aggressively.

The anger from the discovery earlier doesn't cross my mind at all as I think about the lonely apartment he is dropping me off at, especially with the feeling that accompanies the abandonment. I know he won't come back later. This isn't one of those times where I can talk him back into staying at my apartment or coming to pick me back up later to go out. This is one of the few times where my heart sinks so far, so rapidly, that I am at a total loss.

The eyes that always hold some adoration or admonishment are simply like a slate, wiped clean. I cannot see one glimmer of how Jaxx used to look at me. And then the anger comes like a flood, more like a tsunami. I remember the red cap falling to the floor.

"You promised it was only pills!" I shout and snatch my keys from his dangling pointer finger. I don't look at him as he exits the driver's seat and passes me, heading toward the curb.

I don't care how he is getting home.

I don't even look at him as I walk around him like an obstacle. No more words are spoken. I get into the driver's seat and slam the door.

There is no fucking way I'm driving home.

Even though "home" is only a parking lot away from where I am currently, I want him to know how angry I am; I will show him what he has done.

I black out.

Autopilot into the Ghetto

I wake up to drunken laughter, and the darkness startles me. My eyes catch the neon lights of the In-N-Out Burger sign, a familiar landmark in unfamiliar territory.

It is very dark outside. It must be two a.m., and I am in a parking lot somewhere in some part of Los Angeles I've never been.

I slowly remember the fight with Jaxx and puking in the parking lot.

I must have driven here in spite, to get away. Where am I?

Swarms of young, drunk people are walking into In-N-Out Burger. A few of them look over at my car. This is frightening.

My vision is blurry. However, it's more dangerous to stay in this parking lot than to figure out how to get home. At least I'll be a moving target in South Central then.

"God, please help me find the 405, thank you," I pray out loud.

My phone is nowhere to be found. I anxiously reach my fingers along my seat and then stuff them into the small opening between the center console and my seat.

Bingo!

I grab the thin rectangle and pull it up from the crevice.

Shit!

My stomach takes a blow as I see a black screen. My phone is dead.

Shit!

I start to whimper, and a new group of drunk college kids walks toward my car, holding red cups and drunk-chanting, "SC! SC!!"

Oh God! I have a UCLA sticker on my car!

The darkness makes me claustrophobic, and now the crowd of drunk students has found my car a nice target.

I flash my headlights on and off to try to light up the street a bit more as I quickly pull away from the Trojans. It's dark. This neighborhood is not familiar.

How did I get here?

I shudder as I discern two men next to the driver's side door of a beat-up Honda. They watch my car pass, the only car on the street, my charcoal Range Rover sticks out like a Bruin at an SC party.SC party.

I blackout.

I wake up in Jaxx's bed, tucked in. Jaxx is gone.

The Writing on the Wall

My backpack is heavy, crammed with several books, including *Astronomy 101*, several Criterion Shakespeare compilations and a few binders. I struggle as I jump over the low cement wall in front of the gated parking lot. I reach into my back pocket to retrieve the key Jaxx gave me. I exhale as I remember what I saw a few days prior.

According to Jaxx, no one is home, so this should be perfect.
Once inside the apartment, I set up all of my books on the glass living-room table, open my laptop and begin to type out the answers to my boring astronomy review. I hear someone fumbling with the knob and Lexi enters looking surprised.
"Kali! Hi! Is Jaxx here?" Lexi says.
Lexi is Jaxx's roommate, but also a girl I have known since high school. She is a grade above me. She was known as "one of the guys."
"Hey! Sorry! Jaxx said I could study while you guys were out," I say.
"Yeah, totally fine, just haven't seen him in a minute. You are so welcome. Make yourself at home," Lexi says.
"Wait, you haven't seen him?" I ask.
"No, he's been, well, kind of MIA, actually." Hanging up her keys, she continues, "and like he needs to pay rent."

"That's super annoying because he said he was with you and said you needed to give him rent."

She laughs, hard. "Yeah, No. Wow," Lexi says. There is no need to say more. Her laugh says it all, and I know Jaxx.

"I'm worried about him," I say.

"Me too, dude, me too," Lexi says.

She pulls a chair up next to me and slides my books to the left. I close my computer.

"What's going on?" I ask.

My gaze drifts up to the wall to the right of the table.

"WHAT THE!" I shout.

A splash of what is clearly blood is dashed across the upper part of the white wall. I stretch my arm out and point.

Lexi says, "Oh My God. Is that—"

"That is blood, Lexi," I say.

She goes to the kitchen and gets a hand towel wet.

"Kali, Jaxx is not right, right now. He's not himself," she says.

In shock, I watch her stand on a chair and scrub away the streak until the spot is light pink and then gone. My mind races. My entire world has just shifted. And I feel the weight of what has just presented itself as if I have been thrown right into the middle of a centrifuge.

After a short conversation about how we can help him and if we can help him, I pack up my books and leave in a daze.

As the apartment door clicks, I stare in front of me, taking in each part of the hallway as I exit the building, out of Jaxx's broken world for good, for the last time. I am shattered.

I have no recollection of driving back to my aunt's house: lost in times that continue to tear me further and further away from what I planned for myself.

Jaxx told me that he didn't want me to "move to LA, get drunk, and forget about" him. Well, I had done two of those things. The moment he left me alone at my new apartment, I was taken by three different people, believing they were like him. I believed they were there for when he couldn't show me the ropes. Instead of running back to Jaxx to tell him what had taken place, I ran fast and far away, far too ashamed to tell anyone, especially Jaxx. Instead, I said I didn't want any contact with him.

But now, after I finally let Jaxx back into my life and he swooped so seamlessly back into the role of my knight and protector, this.

He helped me move out of my terrible living environment and brought me to live in his. He lay next to me and stroked my head as I battled through my winter finals. He gave me pain medication to help my migraines, back pain and nausea. Now—he has brought the magic into a city I learned to hate, opening my eyes to the dazzling parts of Hollywood. Why did he have to dismantle everything, now? After we have shared lattes and split turkey paninis at our favorite Cafe on Main Street in Venice and taken trips to the Getty Villa so I could complete an extra credit assignment, now that I have fallen so safely back in love with him, he has to go and tear it all down. He has effortlessly destroyed all that I thought was real. Every part of our messed up love story was a lie. He is still the addict; that I have come to understand, but not yet fully accept. I asked him for two things: to be honest about what was going on with him and to tell me if he ever started to use heroin or a needle.

My mind flashes back to every time I questioned his sobriety, looking into a set of eyes that were a little too red or a bit too droopy to have been affected only by playing with pills.

Petiole: January 2010

No wonder her turquoise ring
stayed upon her right hand
ring finger for so many years
until it was taken by a man who drew her in, posing as a new-age version of
her hero.
That man's petiole oil was nothing but a facade—
for he uncovered his boyish ways before she even had time to mention
her interest and why:
his smell, his turquoise-studded bracelet.

DR. SCOTT (MD, G.P., P.C.P.): DECEMBER 29, 2009
Primary Care Visit
Chief Complaint: neck and back pain past year, increased in last six months
S: intense back and neck pain, tension headaches, been going to physical therapy (Ayn Aldo) 2x/week
2 weeks ago SI [suicidal ideation], no SA [suicide attempts], improving at home, anxiety 10 ½ /10
Objective: neck sprain, depression
Assessment/Plan: MDD/Bipolar/GAD, tachycardia with GAD, neck sprain, chronic pain, chronic stress syndrome, x-ray spine
I consent that my doctor, Dr. Scott and FFM (Fuller Family Medicine) can discuss my care with my therapist and psychiatrist.
Signed Kali Rae Wheeler

Losing Control

I watch the different characters walk into the restaurant. I took one of Jaxx's new pills in the car. It was supposed to be stronger than the small Roxicodone he bumped up to from Norco. (See Appendix W.) I also take a Soma. (See Appendix X.) Jaxx always paired the pill of choice with a Soma. I never questioned it. Somas were the cheapest pills, but a good add-on. I often found myself chewing on a couple of Somas out of pure boredom. It is a throw-away drug.

Jaxx had tips and tricks to make the opiates work better. (See Appendix W.) For instance, we never took pills without having an entirely empty stomach. At times, this method made me throw up, but the pills had already hit my bloodstream by the time I started retching. He would pair the pain pills with pills of pure acetaminophen. I would take three to four extra-strength arthritis pills to pump the numbing effect of the cumulative acetaminophen and opioid pair.

He also had another over-the-counter pill to combat the acid that would run through the opioid content quicker. By taking the oxy with one of these stomach-acid-reducing pills, we slowed the ability of our stomachs to breaking down the pill, therefore keeping it in our systems longer.

Tonight, for New Years, Jaxx had taken me to eat at a famous spot in LA. We are both back in Newport Coast for the winter break.

High on pain meds, I feel like everyone in the restaurant is staring at us. And they probably are, to some degree. Jaxx has recently been hanging out a lot with his cousin, Stephen and is benefiting from his cousin's quick rise to fame on a television show.

Stephen is paid huge sums of money to show up at clubs. Jaxx has been tagging along for the ride. However, in tagging along, he was offered a possible job. So, along with modeling, Jaxx has been in talks with a major network about a spin-off show that would film in Hollywood. They even mentioned that I would be a part of the show with a role similar to "the brunette girl in *Entourage*." I've never really understood the premise exactly.

I didn't get my hopes up until tonight, eating in this new place that seems wrought with stardom and fame, dying to start a new life in this amazingly curious city.

Jaxx looks like a model, with his faux-hawk intact and his designer dog tag. I probably look young but am sporting very high heels. I have been so very excited to go out tonight, but he picked me up a bit late. Jaxx has made plans for us to go to two of the clubs that he is promoting.

We will go to the first club, Palihouse, for about a couple hours and then move on to the more hipster Bordeaux. They both have a lounge feel, more than a real dance club vibe, but they are also both very selective about who they let in.

I've never really had to deal with any issues around getting into the "VIP" clubs or whatever you would call them. If you are not a girl, unless you purchase a table or a very expensive bottle of alcohol (I'm talking thousands of dollars here) as well, you don't have a chance getting inside these places. I have always been surrounded by friends who were either promoting the event or working within it (DJs, etc.) Even though the whole thing is a dumb facade, it is still a perk to be let in without issue.

Tonight Jaxx gave me Norco, but he also picked up some 80's, a slang term for Oxycontin. I'm not getting high enough off of the Norco and beg him for a piece of an 80. He sucks off the blue coating as usual. (They don't work if you leave the time release coating on.) This is how I can tell if Jaxx has taken anything, his lips are blue from the coating. Jaxx breaks the pill into quarters. I take a quarter.

Around midnight we make it to Palihouse. We don't celebrate the stroke of midnight. I lose Jaxx somewhere in the darkness of the hallway leading to where we were heading. I suddenly become too nauseated and insecure to stay in the dark and so I head back out toward the parking lot. I don't feel fancy enough to be where all of these seemingly very cool, much older people hung out. I meander outside the club trying to find my balance again. The men working the door, looking important in their matching designer suits and earpieces ask me several times if I am feeling okay.

I black out.

I wake up outside the club, hunched over on a parking hump, staring at the ground. I hear Jaxx, and the thump of his Jack Purcells on the concrete.

"Kali! Babe! Eric just grabbed me; are you okay?" Jaxx asks.

I notice a pair of designer shoes standing directly in front of me.

"Yeah, she's not doing well, Jaxx," a man says. She almost collapsed telling us she was fine. I brought her to sit down, and she fell over."

"Thanks, Kevin. Can you grab me a water?" Jaxx asks.

"Sure thing, boss," Kevin says. I hear his steps on the asphalt.

"Kali, baby, look at me," Jaxx says.

I can't move my head. It's so heavy that it's drooping closer and closer to the pavement.

I try to talk, and my words are jumbled.

I black out.

"Dude, you've got to take her to the hospital," Kevin says.

"She's white, I mean like she's super pale, bro," another voice adds.

"I know, I know," Jaxx says.

He sounds upset.

"Hey, tell Stephen I'll call him," Jaxx says.

Jaxx picks me up like a child. I can feel his legs shaking as he struggles to stand up straight and slowly starts walking.

The security guard, Blake, places a water bottle between my body and Jaxx's chest. I am folded into him.

"Thanks, Blake," Jaxx says.

"Kali, love, you've got to drink the entire bottle," Jaxx says to me. "We are going to go lay down, and be comfortable. Happy New Year, baby!" I feel him kiss my forehead. "You're beautiful. You know that?" Jaxx continues to talk. "Can you tell me what day it is, love? ... Okay, how about what's your favorite band?" He doesn't stop. "Kali! Oh my God! I think I see Dave Matthews!"

I mumble something in response, unable to move my mouth in the right way.

Back in the car, and with help, I drink the entire Fiji bottle. I am finally able to open the iron curtains that have become my eyelids.

Slumped over to the middle of the armrest, I want to tell him so many things, but I can't keep my mind awake. I am unable to think as I become impossibly nauseous and inconceivably dizzy.

I wake up at 2 a.m., my body still folded over the armrest of Jaxx's car. But now, we are moving.

Where are we?

Jaxx is driving, but he doesn't know I'm awake. I don't have the strength to tell him.

"I've taken her pulse every five minutes for the past three hours. She seems fine, but she won't wake up," Jaxx says. His voice is shaking, "I'm on my way right now."

I watch the radio. I don't even wonder why. It's all I can do.

I study the digital numbers and the way they seem to focus and refocus themselves. They are orange, fluorescent rectangles, extending to join the others like a geometric centipede growing against the green background of the clock. The numbers whirl and twist and then refocus themselves.

I stare and listen, acknowledging the present and all of its simplistic complexity. I slowly begin to hear the sounds coming out of the radio. They are distant.

So this is it.

Blackout.

A Fish outta Water

I make it back to Newport Coast after the night back in The Hills with Jaxx. I don't remember how, just being cranky as the midmorning sun gives me an instant headache blaring through the front windshield of Jaxx's truck on our way to the 405 freeway. It's winter break, so I'll be in Newport Coast at my parents until classes begin again.

It is a cold January on the Coast.
I exhale as I slam the door to the Range. I'm about to enter my first meeting of the new year.
A group of men and a few women are standing in front of the steps smoking cigarettes and drinking coffee.
I cannot believe I am back here again.

Before moving forward, I flash back to Jaxx's apartment. Specifically to that first night back together, lying next to one another after being separated shortly after my move to Santa Monica.
I'll never forget that night. We said we would never find anyone that fit as well as we fit together. He gave me a handful of Norcos, and we basked in the fuzziness. All was well. He was my baby blanket. I never felt safer.

And then, flash forward: the red cap bouncing off the laminate floor of his bathroom.

"Jaxx!" I yell, "You swore to me!"

I cried that night before realizing the devastating reality.

And then days after, found out the actual weight of what had just transpired. The fact that I would never be back, after slamming the door behind me that day.

I blink, slowly, back to reality, and have to lean into the next step to muster up the momentum needed to walk into the building. I look down at the mid-thirties surfer-types as they stare at me for being: a) young, b) sad, c) at an Anonymous meeting. Shit. I turn back to my car realizing I've left my *Big Book*.

"Kali!" a man shouts.

No.

How the hell...

I hesitantly turn around. This isn't a prime place to be called out by name, especially when you realize it's a familiar voice. My eyes meet Blaise's.

Huh?!

"Hi, Blaise! How are you?" I say, not thrilled.

"Great, good to see you here," Blaise says in a condescending tone.

Dick. Two can play that game.

"Yeah, you too. I need to get inside...so...good seeing you," I say fluidly.

"Well, it was...good to see you. You look great," Blaise says.

"Yeah! Have a good night," I say overly excited.

Really? Life? Really? Why?!

I take another deep breath and quickly head to the stairwell, so that I don't change my mind. Once upstairs I file like a sardine into the mottled-gray-carpeted room. About thirty plastic white chairs are set up around the perimeter of the rectangular room. I pick a seat with an empty chair next to it and place my book on the chair, my purse, underneath.

"Coffee's ready!" a man shouts behind me. He's far too close to my ears to be shouting.

Not tonight, buddy. Don't f-ing yell.

I carefully get up and step over the seat to grab myself a cup of coffee. Six Splendas ought to do the trick tonight. I'm careful not to make eye-contact with anyone in line behind me. I keep a pleasant but weak smile on my face returning to my chair.

Okay, so, I'm back here again. I'm new. So I'm going have to go through the judgment process once more. They always expect newbies to share.

When you enter an Anonymous meeting, and it is the size of the one tonight, you would think listening would do the trick. But that's not how these meetings operate. You must announce yourself in increments of sobriety, AND they ask each new person, not new to the program, but simply new to their meeting, to introduce themselves and present a brief summary of what qualifies them to be at their meeting.

Trust me; this specific club is like a cult. There are even seniority and cliques. They all know who was not familiar-looking, and they all have drama amongst themselves and their inter-program relationships. The young people sit together and whisper amongst themselves during shares from the guys with thirty, forty, fifty years of sobriety under their belt, who share the same damn stories each time.

The outcasts sit where I am sitting. I want to make it known that I'm not here to chat. At the moment, I truly need healing. And the divine inspiration to ignite within me to make this change occur rapidly.

Tonight's meeting is a long one, three hours. Here's the plan, all mapped out intricately in my mind-world: I am too shy to leave a meeting before it is over and I have spoken to the people who inspired me. So if I get my ass to the meeting, I'm guaranteed to be sober for that three-hour period. no questions asked. So on this chilly evening in January, I mourn the second ending of my very toxic relationship with Jaxx, in a room of thirty-five addicts.

Almost every share has to do with love intertwined with addiction.

Jaxx is different, I think to myself.

He wouldn't have ever laid a hand on me. He was out of his mind drunk when he threw his boot at me. I needed those pills. I was hurting. He was just trying to help me. He is one million times better than the guys in Los Angeles.

I wince as I remember each one in a flash, each one bringing with it a familiarly awful feeling. He would kill those guys if he ever found out. I tear up, reminding myself that he will never know what happened. I blink quickly and stare at the tiled ceiling to keep my cheeks dry.

"And I just thought that if I just kept showing up something would happen...something—" a gray-haired woman says, "and you know what? It did. And today I am thirty-seven years sober, and running toward each day with the zeal I had as a kid."

Clapping erupts around the room.

"It gets easier!" She raises her voice above the clapping. "It works if you work it! And you will find happiness again!"

Yeah, right. Sober I can do, but sober and happy? Yeah right. I'm not made of the same stuff as the rest of this population.

"Even you young faces. You too can do this. You are not too young to be here. Congratulations to you for addressing this before you have truly hit bottom," the woman says.

Okay, fine, I like her.

I hate when addicts in the program mention young people not hitting their true bottom and therefore not being able to recover until they do so. It is such a false accusation. Although I am not homeless, dying, or in a mental institution, I've gotten damn close to the last two on several occasions. And I will only go up from here. There isn't enough time for me to continue down this rotten path.

"My name is James, and I'm an addict. Well…recovering, I guess," a young man says.

"Hiiiii Jaaaaaaaammes," the group replies in unison.

A couple of rebels stretch their words a little longer than the rest.

"Hi James," I mumble, looking down at the *Big Book* I am clasping. My fingers are sweaty as I peel them off to fumble around through the pages.

I look over at James. He is sitting to my left in the far corner, jet black hair swung in front of his face like Justin Bieber. His knees peek through his skinny jeans; he looks young, maybe twenty-five. Leaning forward, James clasps his hands together and speaks while looking at the ground. Occasionally, when James mentions a very intense situation, he looks up as if to say, "Recognize me. I struggled harder than you did. Let's talk more about who used a needle and who didn't because I did. Translation: I am a REAL addict."

He is one of those evangelical drunks.

I study James carefully; I can't grasp his obsession with how his addiction looked on him. He truly seems to feel that it identified him. And this is why I don't enjoy these groups sometimes. With some addicts, their process involves speaking only about where they've been, not where they are headed or where they are in the now.

Addicts is a term used in Alcoholics Anonymous, Narcotics Anonymous, Eating Disorders Anonymous, and other specialized anonymous groups like this one or Christians Addictions. It is an umbrella term for alcoholics, drug addicts, sex addicts, codependents (sometimes). It's not necessary to say, "Hi I'm Kali; I'm an addict, alcoholic." Instead, you just say "Hi, I'm Kali; I'm an addict."

But some people are a bit overly enthusiastic about their name tags and like to name each issue separately.

James is one of these guys.

In these cases, the share can be very detrimental to a newly sober member because it only identifies with the addict in them. I hate these kinds of shares because they turn into a who-fucked-up-worse discussion.

In good meetings, the meeting director will allow each person's share to be the full three minutes, but then make a general comment to the group to remember to stay on topic for today's discussion. The leader of that meeting would announce something like: "If you would like to speak to a sponsor after the meeting about other topics, we would love for you to hook up with one of—raise your hands, sponsors, accepting newbies—these fine people."

I drift off again and see there is a man staring directly at me. He is sitting a few seats away from the speaker. But instead of respecting the speaker or simply looking down into his coffee (normal procedure) he is looking my way.

I catch his glance and look down quickly. Upon returning my gaze to James, I have to tilt my head away from this mans direction to keep from looking straight at this guy.

What are you doing? STOP, creeper!

I get hot inside with anger.

STOP looking at me.

I shift my chair, switch my right leg over my left and reposition my hands. I feel scrutinized. I can't focus. Not that I was tuned into anything, but my own sorrow, aka the words Jaxx spoke to me the day before I moved to Los Angeles in my bedroom in Newport Coast. It's become my mind's habit of reminding me how worthless I am now.

Jaxx's voice echoes in my mind throughout the meeting:

"I just don't want you to move to LA, get drunk and forget about me...

"I just don't want you to move to LA, get drunk and forget about me...

"...move to LA, get drunk and forget about me...

"...move to LA, get drunk and forget...

"...get drunk and forget...

forget..."

I hold back the tears welling up behind my eyelids.

The creepy guy continues to stare at me. He downs his coffee, then looks up at me, maintaining eye contact longer than is socially appropriate. He looks back down into his cup. Then back up at me and smirks.

Damn this guy is a professional.

I am pissed. I catch his gaze intentionally and clench my jaw. Surprisingly, he catches my reaction and points to his coffee and then points to the coffeemaker behind me.

I am super embarrassed and show it on my face. I sink into my chair with a funky smile on my face.

"Oh," I mouth, biting my bottom lip in awkwardness and nodding.

"Break time! We will have a fifteen-minute intermission. Big Books are for sale over in the corner with Pete," the man says.

Pete raises his hand nonchalantly and says, "Coffee will be brewing shortly; does anyone want decaf?"

"No!" several people shout in unison.

Did they practice this?

I remain seated as the rest of the group gets up and socializes, hugging new people and embracing the ones who received chips. I want to remain unseen.

The staring guy appears from behind a couple of people chatting. He doesn't look at me as he passes through the opening in the chairs to my right. He gives me an awkward straight-across emoji face as if I have offended him with my silent accusation and reaches over me to grab a Styrofoam cup. The counter is a few inches from my head.

"You want a cup?" he asks.

Loving his complete lack of interest in me, I look down at my cup. It's almost empty.

"Sure, thank you," I say.

"I wasn't staring at you." He laughs. "So don't flatter yourself. I'm just exhausted."

"Ha! Yeah." I take the cup he's holding out to me.

"I'm guessing you like it black?" he says.

"Am I that easy to read?" I reply.

"No. You just seem sad. And when I'm sad, I don't want shit in my coffee. I just want the caffeine to get me through the meeting," the friendly stranger says. He slides through the opening again and holds out his hand. "Beau."

I fumble around with my book and coffee and manage, "Kali," with an awkward smile.

He sits down in the formerly empty chair beside mine.

"You mind if I grab this seat? It's stuffy over there with all of the old-timers, and I'm going to need more coffee tonight," Beau says.

"Ha, yeah sure. And me too," I say.

Beau reveals that he is a UCLA graduate, works in emergency medicine, like his father, and is from Santa Barbara, where he owns a beach house. He explains that he was pre-med at UCLA and decided not to go to medical school right after graduating, for personal reasons.

His father and brother are doctors and his mother a nurse. He is confident and alluring in his complete lack of anxiety around talking with me. I guess that he's about thirty.

"Alright, please return to your seats. The second part of our meeting starts in two minutes," a meeting director shouts through cupped hands.

Our conversation continues without a break. He says things like: "You looked very sad. I'm not going to ask why because I know that you shouldn't be because you radiate... That's why I had to grab this seat. It looked like you needed a good laugh. And I'm great for that... I think..." he says, waking me.

"Let the meeting commence!" the meeting director shouts a few minutes later.

I look toward the center of the circle attentively as Beau leans over and whispers into my ear, "I wasn't staring at the coffeemaker."

The meeting ends, and Beau walks with me to my car. He explains that he loves going to early morning meetings and that there is one early the next morning.

I flash quickly back into Jaxx's arms and then travel quickly across Dane's living room floor to Aaron's windowsill and Jason's handgun, and return to Beau, an older doctor, (well, basically a doctor, I think and come to believe) who wants to go with me to an early morning Narcotics Anonymous meeting at my favorite church. What else am I going to do except think about what I've ruined and fend for something to take the edge off?

"Yeah, definitely," I say.

"Great. Have a good night, Kali," Beau says.

I get into the Range Rover, the same one that drove me to LA and into so many dangerous situations, the same one that sat outside my sixteenth birthday party before any of this happened.

A new rap album blasts above my thoughts. I speed past the restaurants on Pacific Coast Highway, past the Bay Club, where Jaxx treated me like a princess...UGH!

I turn the volume up louder.

Beau is just a nice person who wants a companion to a meeting. He is not hitting on me. He just wants a friend. It's just a meeting, and it's at six a.m.! No one in history ever asked someone on a "date-date" located inside a church in the morning. He is not hitting on me.

The Serenity Journal

January 15, 2010

Dream last night… A huge truck about as long as three houses with an open top drove by my window as I was standing on the balcony. The truck was filled with dead bodies with only sheets covering their heads. Each had lost an appendage.

XO Kali Rae]
(See Appendices A, G, F, Y.)

DR. FIASCHETTI (M.D., PSYCHIATRIST): JANUARY 20, 2010
Adderall 20-40 mg (See Appendix K.)
Xanax 1 mg (See Appendix B.)
Neurontin 200-400 mg, seemed to work well but led to mania.(See Appendix I.)

January 21, 2010

I admit I am powerless over my disorder and I believe that a power greater than myself will restore me to sanity. A higher power is who placed me in this room along with these other struggling addicts, some of whom who have recovered. I'm back in the program.

Jaxx keeps calling, and I feel deceitful when he says he loves me and I say it back. Sobriety...I am ashamed that I took more Xanax and Ativan than I had intended to today, but I know it's one day at a time and tomorrow things will be different. Tomorrow I will take the prescribed dosage. I have to show I can make it through. Tomorrow will be day one.

I sometimes wonder why I have to struggle so hard to be comfortable in what I'm doing...excuse me, to be accepting of myself. Why did I have to fall head-over-heals with a heroin addict? I know it's not his fault, but Jaxx did provide the drugs for free. I hate knowing that I might break his heart. I'll just take it super slowly, I guess. I can't stand the fact that I felt I could do anything, that I was on top of the world when I was taking opiates. I got straight A's while using. I also despise that Jaxx is attributed to these drugs. Of course, I was in love with Jaxx. I thought everything was perfect. But the entire time I was high. How am I supposed to know what was real and what was fake?

XO Kali Rae

January 22, 2010

Location: Santa Barbara, California—Beau's beach house

    I said I would write every day, so I am doing just that. This song I heard earlier reminded me of Jason. His eyes were the scariest part of the whole thing, aside from the gun. Well, his eyes were worse. He duped me into thinking he was a good guy—impressing me with this love for the church, his job as a physical trainer and his commitment to his schoolwork.

    He came off very mature, and even my mom believed this eighteen-year-old asshole was at least twenty-six. He even talked to my parents when I overdosed [on prescription benzos]. He met my parents! He came to my house. He even went to dinner with my mom, me and Bea, my mom's roommate from college.

    Well, eventually after I had slept with him a few times—big mistake—he took a gun out of his drawer, laughed and then pointed it at me and told me to suck his dick, "bitch." Jason even shot it (w/out a bullet in it of course) to scare me.

    The weirdest thing is, after the fact, he pulled out a Bible and began reading. He looked into my eyes as if he saw right past the fact that I was human. His mind was telling him he was Alpha dog and I was the fucking terrier.

    XO Kali Rae

January 23, 2010

Location: Santa Barbara, California—Beau's beach house
   Panic Attack. God, please help me. Can't do this alone. HELP.
   Certain humiliating memories we tell ourselves ought not to be shared with anyone. They weren't there... He looked at me with these evil eyes and while he was standing in the kitchen said something like: "You're on my bed wearing my shirt... It looks like you're taking over."
   He was very odd—just the way he glared.
   XO Kali Rae
   (See Appendices G, Y.)

The Doctor's Beach House

The entire wall is a window. We are on the second floor of a serene beach house, Beau's home.

I met Beau a couple of weeks ago at my first meeting back in the program. On a whim, I decide to accompany him on a road trip to his beach house. It couldn't hurt, right? I need to get away from Jaxx anyway. And Beau is in the program. I don't have to worry about opiates. It is a fresh, healthy decision, I think, new beginnings, Kali, new beginnings! My subconscious counsels me.

The fact that his beach house is in Santa Barbara also influences my decision. I know the area because it is near a magical place my parents used to take us to as kids. I loved going to Zeke's house in Montecito. Zeke was my father's client, who always stocked the game room when my siblings were kids and got to come to town. It was heaven for us kids. We would fall asleep in the home theater after bingeing on Red Vines and movie popcorn, wake up and carry the kayak across the street to the beach.

I return his text.

Me: Yeah, I'm down

The master bedroom upstairs has a closet the size of my room, or my bedroom and a half. The sound of the waves is enchanting, and the sky is such a gray color it looks like it might storm. The dark blue waves are chaotic with white caps, and they crash into the rocks outside the house like they are smacking into an unwanted visitor. The layered break of the surf lulls me back to sleep.

A male voice shouting hurls me awake. "Beau! Get out of my house, son!" I hear someone stomp up the stairs.

"Oh my God. There's a girl here, honey," an older female voice says to the man.

This must be Beau's mom. She's am emergency room nurse. Beau's father runs a popular practice here in Santa Barbara. He's the area's general physician.

I had been staying in a room separate from Beau's, which I very much appreciated as a gentlemenly gesture, even without hostile old people barging in at seven a.m.

I hear the pitter-patter of feet on the wood stairs, and Beau's mother is now in the doorway.

"Honey, I don't know what you see in my son, but he is not good enough for you. You are too young. You have a bright future ahead of you. Get away from him as soon as possible. He's my son, but he's very sick right now," Mrs. Daus says.

She doesn't waver in her intent to get this message across. She asks no questions of me. Beau's father shows up next to his wife, jutting his shoulder in front of her in the doorway.

Well, he sure is an ass.

"Listen to me and listen well. If you stay with my son, he will steal your medications and take your money. He is a criminal. You should leave now! Cut all ties with him. He's toxic to every single person he comes into contact with. Please listen to me, I'm his father, and I am telling you, stay away from my son," Mr. Daus says.

He's mean, I can tell. But he's honest. It's like they are pleading with me. Their eyes are so fraught with worry, it's shocking.

What has this guy done in his past? What could Beau have done that would cause this sort of reaction?

Dr. Daus is still trying to reach me.

"This guy is not for you. Pack up your things and leave him behind. Have your parents come get you. Hell, I'll pay for a driver. Just get out of this situation while you can," Dr. Daus says.

Beau is shouting something incomprehensible from upstairs, and then I hear his frantic footsteps down the stairs: "Don't talk to her. She's my girl," Beau says in a frenzy.

"She is not anyone's girl. She is her own woman, and she's smart enough to leave you now that she knows the truth!" his mother yells, and breaks into tears, "I've got to wait in the car, I can't handle this, Marty," Mrs. Daus says and exits the room.

"Beau! Get out of my house within the next five minutes, or I will have you arrested," Dr. Daus shouts.

"Oh God, he has drugs, honey!" Mrs. Daus's voice is shaking. She brings a bag of pills into the doorway. "What are these? I know he won't tell me. Will you? I'm not mad. But what are these drugs doing in Marty's home?" Mrs. Daus says.

"I-I, really don't know," I say honestly.

Her voice is lower and now, wobbly, revealing her age, "Oh JEEZUS Christ, Beau. How could you? How could you bring this girl here like this? Did you know he had these too?" Mrs. Daus pulls a new bottle of pills out of her purse. "Come, upstairs, honey. What is your name?" Mrs. Daus asks.

"It's Kali, Mom!" Beau shouts.

"Come with me, Kali," she says, grabbing my hand.

Beau stiff-arms me so I cannot scoot past him up the stairs with his mom.

"I will call the police if you touch her again," Mrs. Daus says and pulls me past Beau, up the stairs, and into what looks like a drug-den.

Beau's suitcases are overturned, and there are paper bags and plastic baggies of pills strewn about next to boxers and ties and nice slacks.

"What are all these?" I ask hesitantly.

I am afraid of speaking in this environment. I don't know who to trust. Beau's dad is still shouting at Beau downstairs.

"I have no idea what's going on; I don't think. Beau said that this was his house," I say. "I'm so sorry for the confusion. I'll leave right away. I'm so sorry," I start crying, and Mrs. Daus pulls me into her.

"It's okay, let's get you home," Mrs. Daus says.

"Mom! Don't touch her!" Beau is yelling from outside the room at the top of the stairs. Now he is charging toward us. He's back! It's like *The Shining*. "Kali, they're lying to you! Don't listen!" Beau shouts.

Beau pulls us apart. His mother lets out a gasp and turns around when I see Marty charging through the door just as his son did a few moments earlier.

"Don't you EVER touch her again! I'm warning you, Beau!" Dr. Daus shouts.

I run out of the room unaware of my surroundings or who I'm with and only focused on running far away from whatever this is becoming. There's going to be a fight.

I hear Dr. Daus shout, "This is my house you piece of shit, you worthless piece of fucked-up potential. You disgust me. You disgust me so much I wish you weren't my son. GET OUT!"

Ultram

"What are those?" I ask.

Beau and I are in a motel parking lot. He has to pick something up from a friend. I haven't asked him where we will be staying tonight. I haven't said a word to him. Not since the fight with his parent.

Beau found me about a mile down Pacific Coast Highway shortly after I ran away. I wasn't ready to leave the city like his dad suggested. I didn't want my parents to be right. I planned to gather my thoughts, while getting further and further away from the toxic situation that was Beau.

However, it wasn't long before Beau pulled up behind me. My neon orange backpack didn't help the getaway, nor did the fact that I walked on the one paved road out of the beach town. I hesitantly succumbed to his sweet talk and got in his Mercedes Benz before I manage a better plan.

"Ultram," Beau says. (See Appendix N.)
"What are they for?" I ask.
"Getting off of opiates," Beau says.
"Can I try one?" I ask.
"Yeah, sure, they're sour, though," Beau answers.

I stick a triangular pill in my mouth, and my gag reflex kicks in right away. I retch and regain composure.

"Yeah, they're pretty ba—" I say. I can't even talk. It is that bad. Whoa, it's numbing my mouth as it dissolves. It's like eating bile that has the effects of Novocain. I have chewed many kinds of pills, but Ultram? That is a skill. To keep from vomiting is a skill with that drug. It is awful.

"So you're not a doctor?" I ask.

"No," Beau answers, "I got kicked out of EMT school. I was in a sober living house in Newport when I met you."

"Damn. That's why you're looking for a job?" I ask.

"Yes," Beau says.

"So this is your dad's beach house," I say.

"Yes. The beach house is my father's," Beau says. "If you ever need pain meds, I can use my dad's physician number. I used to do it all the time." Beau is still not looking at me, but is speaking like a sociopath.

"You just call the pharmacy and order them?" I ask.

"Yeah, it's easy. I just pretend to be my dad. I sound just like him on the phone," Beau says.

"Have you ever used a needle?" I ask.

"I was an EMT. Of course, I've used a needle—Oh...no. Not for drugs," Beau says.

"Have you ever done drugs other than pills?" I ask.

Please say no, please say no, please say no.

"No. No needles," Beau says.

Okay, well that's a plus. At least I don't have to worry about catching diseases.

I have a panic attack, in a picturesque beach house, with a guy I think is a doctor, whose parents have just told me to stay far, far, away from him. I am still intrigued. Because that's how it works, I guess... Or maybe just how a brain works on drugs. I am set on this doctor being a great guy, and so when he isn't, I continue painting my illusion of him. I refuse to believe the situation is as bad as it is and give in to it all instead. (See Appendix N.)

January 30, 2010

Help me.
XO Kali Rae
(See Appendix I.)

DR. DAUS (M.D.): JANUARY 31, 2010
Urgent Care Visit
Chief Complaint: flank pain
S: kidney pain with multiple kidney stones. (See Appendix E.)
A/P: ER if worsens or fever remains, Rx Avelox (See Appendix M.)

Pure Whites: January 2010

Sitting around a table,
watching candles flicker slow.
Whisping through the stagnant air,
only 7 of the 8 candles still aglow,
desperate for the oxygen
to sustain them.

Ignorance is bliss if you're not a candle.
With each breath in and each breath out,
waxy life stolen by our blood-sucking veins.

One moment later, another falls black.
Now it's 6 out of 8.
Harder now with each loss,
to imagine the illumination ever coming back.

Hope dwindles as the room fills with doubt.
5 out of 8 candles burn bright,
but then another candle falls victim to the night,
by nothing more than another person's careless sigh.

As the number grows,
the angels come quickly.
They are weak on arrival as well.
They try to spark the dark wick,
to bring the light back to the night,
but another breath steals it quick;
another life of an illuminating pure white.

Now half the candles cease to flow.
The promise of another way,
the promise of another day,
sucked away by the loss of flames.

One can announce the glass half full
but the feeling remains buried
And it throbs deep: it throbs slow.

A change in perspective,
only a Band-Aid for the mess of the artificial reality bringing upon death.

It's too late for any true light to ignite.

As the wax spills forth—
dripping melodically over its cheap enclosure,
one by one, two by two,
they bury the possibility of our false reality transforming into truth.
Watching and waiting for the last flicker to wail,
it's difficult to believe in living when even candles burn out unwillingly

Black Or White: February 8, 2010

To me, love is black
or it's white.
And you've never,
not once,
not ever,
made anything out of this mess of color,
just haphazardly mixed it all together.

So I'm gonna leave.
No,
I'm going to run
as fast as I can away from this frenzy,
away from whatever this is that you've mashed together.

This time,
this part,
is not mine.
This is not mine.
You were a doctor;
fix me.

NCPD: The Courage to Speak Up

It's time now.
"I want to go to the police station," I say.
Beau looks up from his phone, "Okay, are you—"
"Just drive me to the station, I need to report a couple things," I say, sure of myself.

My entire life has been shifted up to this day because of what this man did. Blaise was eighteen, and I was only fifteen. And, after moving to Los Angeles, I've found that my inability to catch the signs of these predators, led me right into the lion's den time and time again.
If they did it to me, they've done it to other people. And I am not okay with sitting here allowing a criminal to ruin another women's life, the way he ruined mine. The fact that these men think they have the right to take advantage of someone when they are not conscious is beyond me as well. I'm not ready to sit in silence with this burden for the rest of my life.

"You okay?" Beau asks from the driver's seat.
"Yeah, I'm good. I've been here before…" I laugh. "To pick up Jaxx."

I walk up the steps toward the regal-looking building, "Newport Coast Police Station," it reads. I realize that I've never actually been inside the building. The Porsche dealership next door drowns out any notions of what's going on inside the police station.

The station is glorified in my mind. Whenever I went to pick up Jaxx, he would come down the steps of this building looking cool as ever. It is a place of unlimited possibilities to me.

For instance, when Jaxx was charged with possession of narcotics and two other small crimes, being drunk in public and urinating in public (or something similar), he came back from that place with nothing to show for it. He was sure he'd get at least a few months in jail. But, Voila! Nothing happened. This place is magic.

Whoa, it's nice in here.

My boots hit the marble floor, and it reminds me of a grand hotel. Once within the actual station, I feel a bit more intimidated. The plastic chairs are stark in contrast to the white walls. There isn't much here.

After I tell the woman behind the glass wall that I want to talk with someone, she questions me. When I refuse to explain in front of the audience of the waiting room, she rolls her eyes and tells me to take a seat. A couple of men are waiting with me. I'm guessing they are waiting for different reasons than mine.

…maybe reasons like crime, real crime.

My mind taunts me.

…since this is a police department, Kali.

A tall, doll-like officer comes in through the wooden doors; his uniform looks pristine, and I wonder if he is the model for the department, or maybe the guy they use in the D.A.R.E. (Drug Abuse Resistance Education) Program commercial. Everyone was in love with our school's D.A.R.E. officer, me included, but Emma's mom was the worst…

"Miss? Would you come this way?" the officer asks. I am shaken back into reality by his cold voice.

The officer leads me into a white room. He asks me to sit at the round, white table, surrounded by the same plastic chairs that were in the waiting area.

"Why are you here today?" he asks after taking the seat opposite me.

"Well—" I start.

By the end of a few minutes, I've forgotten everything I said. My palms are pressed up against one another, slid between my thighs, arms in almost, a diving position. My shoulders are up to my ears. The color has drained from my face, I'm sure.

I need water.

Telling My Story

Mid-confession, the sterile cop, face permanently unreactive, keeps questioning me like an attorney. He questions me exactly the way my father would. But it is tearing me to pieces. Out of nowhere, I begin to burst at the seams, sobbing.

"No! I didn't!" I shout.

"Let me get my partner," he says.

My tears have formed a fish-eye lens. Staring down at my legs, I blink, over and over, trying to focus my mind, pleading with myself to:

1) Hold it together.

2) Go back in time and erase this entire thing.

3) Run. Fast. NOW!

A new officer enters.

"Whoa, whoa..." he says like a father, looking over at Cop Bob, who is now standing in the corner. "Bring us a tissue box, will ya? What did you do to her?"

He takes a seat after placing a single sheet of printer paper in front of me, and a black sharpie. "Relax, everything is okay. I need you to write down the names. Then you're done."

"No!" I say, much louder than I planned. "I'm sorry, it's just, he didn't even believe me."

The first officer enters with a tissue box, still expressionless. The officer says nothing as he places it on the white table and returns to his stance: legs apart, hands in fists, arms crossed. Why is he treating me like a criminal? "He's mad at me. I didn't want to come in here." I don't even know what I'm talking about anymore.

"Listen, Sweetheart, my partner here did alert me to what you told him, and I need some information to take the necessary steps forward," the officer says.

"No." My voice quivers. "I just—No. I just…No!"

I am devastated and now, basically, hysterical. I relived each one of the incidents for the first officer. Now I am confronted with more intense seemingly unrelated questions. This all makes me feel completely worthless, and on top of that, guilty. I am sure it isn't his intention, but I am totally unprepared to do an excavation of my assaults.

I always thought telling my story would be enough.

As the new cop speaks, I tune him out completely. I look down at my wrists.

What would happen if I slit these later? Would it work?

"I don't want to do this anymore," I say, mumbling aloud.

"Do what?" the new officer asks.

"I'm sorry, I've got to go," I say.

"Please just write down their names," he says.

"I can't. I'm sorry. Can I please go now?" I plead. I break down when I catch the other officer in the doorway still looking like a brick wall.

"Just wait a moment," the officer says.

"Let me go now. Please! I don't want to be here!" I shout.

Hold it together, Kali.

"You can't keep me here!" I shout.

Great, Kali, now you're full-on hysterical. Perfect. Totally not crazy.

"I just want to go home," I say.

"But you were underage on at least one of these accounts. You were a minor. They were adults. They assaulted you, Kali," the cop says.

"Please let me go home," I say.

"Here's my card and some information on where to get help. And, Miss?" the new officer says.

He slides the papers over to me on the table and then waits for me to look up at him. "Please look at me," he says.

I glance up reluctantly.

"We want to help you. Please call us when you feel better. We can help you. None of these incidents are your fault," he says.

I look up quickly, a reflex in reaction. I am caught off guard by this simple sentence.

He says it again. "They are not your fault at all."

Beau is waiting in the parking lot of the police station. I am silent on the drive home to my parents. Beau asks a couple of stupid questions that I refuse to acknowledge. My stomach is in my throat, and no one is on my team.

Once home, I charge past Beau into my house. My mother and father are standing by the door.

"Kali, did you really just go to the police station?" my mom asks accusingly as I pass her.

I'm livid, but these reactions keep making me feel like I've just committed a crime.

Slamming the door to my childhood bedroom, I am so angry I could explode. I can hear the three of them, my dad, mom, and Beau talking: my mother's "talking shit" tone is in full effect. She chuckles in the low tone of voice that I know so well. It's usually accompanied by a hand on the forehead and a shaking of her head. She'll then dramatically look up from under her palm, to make this weird inhaling noise, rolling her eyes in the process. I can also hear Beau responding to her without much emotion.

I want to disappear.

How can I be feeling this bad about something that was supposed to fix what happened?

I slide down the door, making it clank against its hinges.

I didn't ever realize until now that the cliché—sliding down the door in a mess of tears while ugly crying—is based in reality. When emotions are so overwhelming that they buckle your knees, it forces you to find the nearest wall to stabilize yourself as you crumple.

He Laughs at My Jokes, Drives, and Supports Everything I Do and Say/ I Don't Have Time to Say No to That

"I want to get a puppy so bad," I whine to my older, wiser, I'll-do-anything-to-make-you-happy boyfriend.

"What kind?" Beau asks.

"A pit bull. I've been looking a long time, and I want to prove the stereotype wrong. They are very loyal dogs," I say. I scroll down the web page of a pit bulls shelter. "I looked at greyhounds too. They're like cats. The problem is, if you let them off the leash they run until their heart bursts."

"What!?" Beau says.

"Serious. Once they're done racing, they're sent to the pound. It's like the trainers just use them up and throw them out. Awful, just awful," I say.

"We could keep it in the house." Beau says.

Beau neglects the one most important aspect of that statement: the house. He doesn't have one. He is currently staying at my parents' house. He told me he wanted to find a place in LA. My parents kindly offered up our extra room in the meantime.

"Let's get a pit. Let's just do it. I want to get you a puppy," Beau says.

Neglecting all surrounding circumstances, I throw my arms around his neck, "Thank you, thank you! Can we go after my class tomorrow?!"

"Yes, baby. Whatever you want. I'll try and find the best place to go," Beau says.

"No, I wanna help! I have to write this Victorian essay," I say. I mock gag dramatically because the Victoria era sucks. (I'm a Romantics person.) "But I want to look with you."

"Whatever you want. You look beautiful in those glasses; I could stare at you all day. But...I won't, because that's creepy. And I'm going to grab the dry-cleaning. Do you want Pete's?" Beau asks.

"Yes! Almond milk latte please!" I answer.

"Okay, get back to writing," he says.

I smile warmly from my fortress of down comforter lined with literature textbooks filled with Old English phrases and cover designs that say outright "You're Going to Hate This Thick-Ass Paperback" *Encyclopedia of Boring Poetry*.

He likes me in glasses. And he's getting me a puppy.

AND a latte...

AND, wait for it, the guy's a doctor? I'll take it.

CORRECTION I thought he was a doctor, but I do not seem to understand it is all a lie.

The next day, sure enough, after turning in the essay I'd worked all night on, Beau shows up in his old black BMW, rocking Ray Bans and looking entirely too important to be picking up a silly college girl. He is on his Bluetooth, looking doctor-like.

"Hey, babe," Beau says, "How was class? Damn, I remember classes here." He leans over to kiss me on the forehead, but I cringe, moving my head away.

"Ugh, that teacher is a Nazi about staying on topic. It's like...I'm a poet, cha dig,'" I say. It makes him laugh. Add: he laughs at my jokes.

He is funny, confident, smart and aggressive. And now that I know more about body language, he is always sitting like an asshole: knees wide, arms-crossed.

"Let's Get a Puppy"

We pull up to the pound. It is as authentic as one would ever think a pit bull-specific pound would be; I chose this dog pound because it was specifically a kill-shelter, meaning they euthanize the dogs if they are not adopted within a set time span (usually a week) of their arrival. And they have a pair of black pit bull puppies abandoned by their mother. The man on the phone last night said that they only have a couple of days left.

Walking up on the gravel outside the cement block of a building, we hear the howls and angry guard-dog-like barks.
"Damn," Beau says.
He grabs my hand. I toss it away.
"Yuck," I say, half kidding, "Yeah this is nuts."
A man in galoshes carrying a mop asks, "Can I help you?"
He sounds pissed. He must think we got lost. My Mark Jacobs purse might look a bit much with my Chanel glasses and designer jeans. I'm wearing UGG boots too…yikes. Beau is no better.
"I called last night regarding a black pit bull puppy," I say.
"We've only got pit bulls," he says annoyed. I look at him eager to hear more. "Just come with me, not sure if we still got 'em, there were two of them, but they've been here a while."

My boots clomp annoyingly, and the buckles clink echoes through the cement hallways. It is like a prison. I've never been, but I imagine this is like a prison. Another guy in galoshes is throwing a bowl of kibble into the cage of a vicious, barking dog. He's jabbing a pole in and out of the cage, probably fighting back the snarling animal.

I see a white-and-black-spotted dog lying in the very back of the narrow cement den.

"Beau, stop. Come look at this one," I say.

"You don't want her; she's sick," the guy in galoshes says.

"We could make her well!" I say.

"No, she has rabies. She'll be euthanized tonight," the man in galoshes says.

"Got it," I say.

I must look noticeably sad from then on because the man all of the sudden becomes hospitable. He even turns around when he speaks to us.

The moment I see Stella and her brother I melt. There are several puppies in the cage, but the two of them stand out. One is jumping all over the other.

"If you want, I can let you guys in," the man offers.

"No way, man. I'm good," Beau says.

"Sorry about the smell. I can rinse the dogs off for you," the man says.

"I wanna go! Let me in!" I say.

The kennel worker laughs and opens up the metal enclosure. One of the puppies bounds forward, stepping in poop on the way. The man scoops the puppy up just in time. He brings him back to me all clean.

"Thank you! Thank you! Thank you!" I shout.

The little puppy is doing circles in the space between my legs on the ground. A very hyper dog.

Beau is busy checking out a couple dogs the next cage over.

"Hey, there's a lab over here!" Beau says.

Enthralled by the squirming puppy in my lap I don't respond. But when I turn to see where Beau is, my gaze falls upon another puppy. She's in a ball, shaking like a leaf in the corner.

"I apologize for the smell," the helpful man says again. "I'd get that one." He points toward the scared puppy.

"Really? Why?" I ask.

"The way she acts. Those are always the better dogs. The one you've got there, he's gonna be trouble. I can tell," the man responds.

I walk into the holding cage to visit with her, but the man saves me again, swooping her up before I can.

"Gimme one second," he says.

"This is the one. I'm telling you. You should get that one. She won't be here long," he says, handing me the now clean, wiggling puppy. "Maybe not even until tomorrow. People don't like the black ones. So we get rid of 'em quick. We have to." I laugh thinking he's kidding. "It's because they don't photograph well. Listen, we're closing soon, and we take care of neutering upstairs. If you want to take her, you should take her now. They probably won't let her stay another day. She's too nervous around people. People who come here aren't looking for that. They're looking for a fighter."

"Is that the one you want?" Beau asks.

"Yes! Oh my gosh!" I shriek. "She's perfect!"

"I'll let you take her for half price, and she can be the last dog they do today upstairs. If you come back at six o'clock she should be all ready to take home," the man says and laughs, scooping up the puppy once more and pushing the other puppy back into the cage. "By the way," the man adds, "This isn't technically a pit bull. It's a Stafford terrier mix." He's reading the label off of the cage. "You still want it?"

"Yes! We want her!!!" I shout.

As we drive home, the four-month-old puppy lies in my arms like a newborn. Her hair is patchy in several places, and she is limp from the anesthesia, but the way she walks is like a pony. I'm instantly in love.

"Stella, because you're beautiful! That will be your name," I say to the newly shampooed puppy.

"Does your mom know?" Beau asks.

Not the pit bull part, rather the Stafford terrier mix part.

"Yeah, my mom knows. But I have to find a place soon. She can stay at your house, too, maybe?" I ask.

Stella will stay with my parents until I find a new apartment big enough to fit Stella and me in Los Angeles or until Beau moves into to his place, which is supposedly within the next couple of weeks.

DR. SCOTT (M.D.): MARCH 29, 2010
PRIMARY CARE VISIT
Chief Complaint: skin lesions on legs
S: boyfriend has MRSA
General: anxious
A/P: folliculitis Rx Clindamycin, Bactroban, hydrocortisone cream. Pt [patient] [educated, rr [relative risk of] MRSA and contagious from carriers

Don't F*** with My Brother

It's a beautiful, Newport morning, clear as ever.

Beau is smoking a cigarette.

"Close the door if you're going to be smoking," Isaak says, irritated, and walks into the kitchen.

Beau gets up and shuts the screen door.

"Bro, did you seriously just fucking blow smoke into my house? Are you fucking kidding me, dude!" Isaak says.

I didn't watch Beau close the screen. But Isaak would not have made that up.

"Huh?" I say confused.

"No. I just closed the door like you asked. Relax…bruh," Beau adds the "bruh" at the end, mocking Isaak.

"You are in my house. So shut the fuck up or get the hell out." Isaak is now standing in the doorframe. His chest puffed out, he is looking directly at Beau, who is not moving an inch back.

I jump up from my seat.

"Guys! Guys! Stop. Beau! Isaak!" I shout and grab Beau's shoulder to pull it back. He resists and swings his arm forward again. I look at Isaak. His gaze is unwavering, like a hawk on prey. "Isaak, he didn't try to blow smoke in the house," I cry.

"Oh yeah, Kali? Really? So I just imagined the cloud of smoke come into my house. He needs to get the fuck out," Isaak says. Isaak inches closer to

Beau. I'm ready to cover my eyes. I've seen Isaak knock someone out on my behalf before and it's terrifying.

"Guys! Whoa, slow down. What's going on?" my dad shouts. He's coming from the entrance to the family room, breaking up the fuming tension almost immediately. I hear sleepiness in his voice, and I squint to see inside. He's wearing his pajamas still. He must have just walked downstairs.

"Sorry, Mr. Wheeler. Isaak here thinks I blew smoke into your beautiful home. But I did not," Beau says.

"Beau, shut up," I say quickly without thought.

"Get out, dude," Isaak says and then backs away, realizing that it is a waste of time to knock Beau unconscious.

> **DR. FIASCHETTI: APRIL 21, 2010**
> Adderall 20mg—manic. (See Appendix K.)

Dr. Fiaschetti, M.D. (Psychiatrist)

Dr. Fiaschetti never ran any tests on me before prescribing this highly addictive drug. She notes simply: "because siblings did well on it."

If I am manic when prescribed Adderall, why would you keep me on Adderall? It would only make sense that a stimulant, especially in combination with the antipsychotics, anti-epileptics, and antidepressants (SSRIS and MAOIS) would send me into overdrive. Not to mention the serotonin syndrome clearly reported when combining a stimulant with any other psychotropic medication. The Promises Treatment Center wrote an article titled "Amphetamine's Role in Serotonin Syndrome." See the excerpt below:

> In combination with other drugs or medications that boost serotonin levels, amphetamine and amphetamine-based substances are known contributors to the onset of severe serotonin syndrome ... In addition to SSRIs, SSNRIs, and MAOIs, substances that can trigger extreme problems when used simultaneously with amphetamines include the opioid medications meperidine (demerol) and tramadol (ultram), the anti-anxiety medication buspirone (buspar), the bipolar disorder medication lithium, the herbal supplement St. John's wort, the synthetic supplement l-tryptophan, and the hallucinogenic drug LSD. (Promises 2017)

And, if it wasn't the Adderall causing me to become manic, the Rifampin I was prescribed for the random MRSA infection I got from my scary boyfriend, causes "schizophrenia-like" symptoms as well as delusions, hallucinations and, of course, SEROTONIN SYNDROME. (See Appendix G.)

DR. FIASCHETTI: MAY 05, 2010
Lamictal 20-50mg—eventually 125mg. Didn't think Lamictal was helping and stopped. (See Appendix P.)
Started again w/Adderall 20-40mg.. (See Appendix K.)
Depakote ER 125mg—increased to twice daily [250mg] "better than Lamictal, no migraines and more like myself." (See Appendix Q.)

Fooled: This Definitely Isn't Dave Matthews.

Beau Daus: the guy who faked being a doctor at an AA meeting, and then, faked owning a beach-house, and then even faked being a paramedic, and sober, also contracted MRSA. Don't ask me how: I have no fucking clue. And I still do not want to think about the letter he wrote Dr. Scott after I relayed to him what my parents had told me about how odd Beau acted at the doctor.

Not only did he act like a psycho, sweating, red, like a fucking guy you wanna punch, he handwrote a long letter apologizing to Dr. Scott for acting weird: "if I did in any way," was the gist of the letter.

At the time he had sores, so we both, of course, had to go to the doctor to be checked. I had a weird mark that was overlooked, written up on the charts as an ingrown hair. But, it grew and grew, until it multiplied and I came to my senses, realizing that all of the drawing salve and A and D ointment in the world, carelessly slopped over the marks, wasn't going to heal something that hadn't healed in months.

I was put on not only oral antibiotics, but also ointment that had to be put up the nose every several hours.

I had to get the original "ingrown hair" drained: There were two spots right between my butt cheeks and another right below my butt that Dr. Scott got to get all up in.

My entire family had to take the mandatory antibiotics for the potentially fatal flesh-eating, staph infection that my wonderful drug-addict, liar friend had given us.

He was kicked out of my house for stealing my medications

I am so intent on getting straight-A's, that I don't pay attention to what Beau does, or how he acts, outside of taking me anywhere I want to go, at anytime, and telling me I am the most incredible thing he has ever seen, or known.

I pay attention when he writes poetry about me and tells me I am too smart for the class that is swamping me. He has a way…or I am a drugged-out narcissist.

In the beginning, I accompanied Beau to hospitals and to fire houses, so he could interview for positions. He never got one position, and later, I would learn it was probably due to the fact that he stole the medications they used to save people's lives and, instead, took them to get high.

He would actually set up IVs for himself. So no, the well-spoken UCLA doctor I'd met that lonely night at that Newport AA meeting, was in fact, none of that. After my father presented me with the gift of picking which Dave Matthews show we could go to, Beau even decided that he would take me to a behind-the-scenes festival where Dave Matthews would be playing.

He then retracts, "I think it's just like the guitar player."

"Oh my god! Tim!" I say.

"Or the guy with the dreads," Beau says.

"Oh my God! Boyd!" My voice higher this time.

My Dad steps in to ask, "Where is this thing?"

"It's in Ventura," Beau says.

My mother pulls me aside in the kitchen before I leave on my "private Coachella" event weekend.

"You know, it's really unlikely Dave Matthews will be there," she says.

"I know. I think it's Tim," I say.

I have no idea that it is all a lie.

At the venue, which is far from Coachella-like, Beau admits, "I think one of the guys may have toured with them once, or for like one show or something… I brought Opana for us!" (See Appendix R.)

"He did get you through your classes," my mom reminds me years later. I am so focused on studying that I leave to Beau stuff like food, travel, sleep. Beau drives me everywhere, brings me food, makes me laugh and tells me I am the best thing since sliced bread.

"Please Recount Those"

"No. Please count them in front of me. Last time I was told I got ninety. I was finished with them a week and a half early! It's not like I took like six pills each day!" I say to the pharmacist behind the counter.

"I'm sorry, ma'am. I'll make a note to count them out each time. Just give me one minute. We count several times before preparing them for pickup. It's very rare for there to be a miscount," the pharmacist says.

She walks between the aisles of white bottles of different sizes. I watch her speak with a white coat. The taller woman in the longer lab coat shakes her head. She looks at the bottle carefully and kind of shrugs as she hands the bottle back to the pharmacist and continues to tell her something. The pharmacist nods nervously. I look at Beau, who is right beside me.

"What idiots," Beau says.

"Relax," I say, embarrassed.

A line has formed behind the "Stand Behind This Line" sign.

The pharmacist returns with the bottle and a little white funnel device. "Sorry for the wait. Yes we will make a note from now on to count them in front of you," she says.

"It's just frustrating because I paid for a thirty-day supply. And then I feel like I've done something wrong when obviously it's not me," I say to her.

"You guys should count them every time," Beau chimes in.

Why are you talking, Beau? We've talked about this: you NOT talking I mean.

"Sir, we count them multiple times. That's why the number is circled on the bottle," the pharmacist says.

She holds up the little orange bottle displaying the circled "90" on the bottom right corner.

"Sorry," I say to her.

"Whatever," Beau says and walks away.

Thank God.

I watch the woman funnel ten by ten into the orange bottle. The device for separating and funneling makes this process very quick.

"Ten." She pauses to let me count. "Twenty," pausing again, "thirty…forty…fifty…sixty…seventy…and…eighty…and ninety," the pharmacist says, swiftly scooping up the pills into the funnel.

"Thank you for checking," I say.

"No problem. Have a great day," she says and hands over a folded white paper bag holding the prescription.

I cringe as I turn around to find a dozen people in line. "Sorry," I mime and quickly head for the exit.

The Serenity Journal: In Not So Serene Times

Writing to You from Sunny, Santa Barbara, California

I'm in Santa Barbara with Stella. Beau and I planned to stay in Beau's mom's house for the weekend. She works as a nurse, so she works from the afternoon through the night and then returns home to sleep all day. Beau got kicked out of my house for stealing my medication, so we alternate between hotels, rather motels, and his mom's house in Santa Barbara. Unbeknownst to me, Beau's mom did not want Beau to stay there. Shortly after we arrive, she finds him sleeping in his old room and kicks him out. I was out walking Stella when I got the news.

June 19, 2010

Just to let you know, I am dying to leave this bullshit. I am at a random motel again with Beau, but this time I had to pay. He acts like he's messed up on something, and I know he didn't sleep last night. He had me try on engagement rings. I hate the fact that I cannot wait to take my next Ultram. Until then, wish me the best!

I've had too much, way too much. Please help me get out of here. I drive me insane. What is love if you don't love yourself? I don't know. Many have taken the unfinished "The Fall of Hyperion" as something disposable, or simply regard it as a failure. This could not be further from the truth. Keats was not out of his mind while composing this. He was out of strength to battle his demons. I'm going to listen to Billie Holiday.

XO Kali Rae
(See Appendices N, P, Q, W, R.)

We Could: June 20, 2010

Why do my memories
Slip away so suddenly?
Why am I left in the dark?
Why do these voices keep telling me to get a move on?
I'm crying alone in my sleep
And I'm lost, I'm lost without you
Without someone to hold me an call me Baby
But the thought
The thought of you and me together
Only comes unnaturally
I know we could make it
We could sort this mess out.
Just tell me you'll pull some weight.
I don't want to have to doubt.
Because I'm lost when you're not around.
And I fall faster when I watch you sink down.
How bout we pull ourselves off the ground, or maybe pull the trigger.
You gotta hold me down,
Because I'm a sprinter.
And I don't want to become your heart's splinter.

DR. SCOTT: JUNE 22, 2010
PRIMARY CARE VISIT
MRSA Rx: rifampin 300 bid [twice per day], call mother to warn about decreased effectiveness of Seroquel and Lamictal, Bactrim d/c [discontinued] N/V [nausea/vomiting]
FOLLOW UP: 1 DAY

Rifampin: Night Terrors, Near-Psychosis, Dementia

The medicine I am prescribed to treat the MRSA infection I contracted from my boyfriend at the time, Rifampin, makes me even crazier than I already am. I have hallucinations accompanied by night terrors, the inability to tell what is real from what is a delusion or even hallucination. I cannot sleep, and when I sleep I have night terrors.

Beau, utilizing his background in medicine, has to care for me like a patient when I wake up screaming multiple times per night, unable to catch my breath, with a fever and an incredibly high pulse. There are moments of this in Newport as well as in Santa Barbara.

When I close my eyes at night, I literally see a nightmare; when I open my eyes to find safety, I cannot decipher what is part of the dream and what is part of reality. It is terrifying.

There are numerous reports of serotonin syndrome as well as people suffering from schizophrenic-like symptoms accompanying the use of Rifampin, one patient noted. This is such a frequently occurring effect of Rifampin that there are multiple articles about it. (See Appendix L.)

How the heck did Beau contract MRSA, anyway? The only time he was away from me is when he told me he was going to attend a special meeting in Long Beach. The evening he came back, he was acting even stranger than usual, sweating, super energetic, annoying, eyes-bulging, but I was too busy studying for an exam the next day to really look into it. Plus, there was nothing I could do, nor wanted to do, to try and figure him out. I just wanted him to take me to class in the morning and be done with it.

DR. SCOTT: JUNE 23, 2010
PRIMARY CARE VISIT
Chief Complaint: flu
S: reaction from abx [antibiotics]
O: MRSA, bipolar (stable)
A/P: cont. abx Rifampin + Bactrim
F/U: 2 days

DR. SCOTT: JUNE 25, 2010
PRIMARY CARE VISIT
Chief complaint: quick wound check
S: pt, reports poor tolerance of current abx for MRSA Currently taking Bactrim and Rifampin po. [by mouth] however, c/o [complains of] nausea and gi [gastrointestinal] complaints. Also reports dizziness.
O: MRSA, bipolar
A: pt. poorly tolerating Bactrim (sulfa allergy) and c/o nausea and disorientation on med. Abscess healing well. Decrease in pain. Pt has increased bp [blood pressure], suspect to a degree stress/anxiety of visit.
P: d/c Bactrim 20g med allergy/adverse side effect Rx Doxycycline 100mg x 14 days, cont. Rifampin as rx'd prescribed, follow.

DR. SCOTT: JUNE 28, 2010 (TELEPHONE)
Mode of contact: Telephone
ADD: access healing, abx reported n/v [nausea/vomiting] cont. doxycycline 100mg

Breaking Up/The Bayfront Proposal

Beau is driving up from Ventura to drive me to dinner, and all I want to do is puke and sleep. I throw on my default "going out last minute" RucKus dress, moaning the whole time.

"Mom I don't wanna go at all," I say.

"Be ready, Kali, that's all I have to say," my mom says from the living room.

"STAWWP," I moan, "I feel like shit."

"Oh my God. Oh my God, Kali. He is in a suit," my mom relays.

"Who cares," I say with little energy.

My plan stands; tonight I will break up with Beau because we are already broken up in my mind, and I hate him.

He gave me MRSA, took me to a fake Dave Matthews Band festival to give me Opana, stole my medication and blamed it on me for being an addict, oh, and did I mention that he tried to commit insurance fraud after a fender bender in my Range Rover? After all of that, plus the fact that he never got an apartment and is NOT a doctor, I have decided to finally look back upon the things my parents had told me: to ask myself why I would ever want to be with someone, even as a friend, who did these things.

"So, I thought we'd go to your favorite restaurant," Beau says from the driver's seat.

"Oh God, Beau. No. You're kidding right?" I say. He's about to take me to the spot Jaxx and I frequented. But Jaxx was the reason I loved it.

"Well I made a reservation," Beau says.

"Whatever," I say, too tired to fight.

I told him ONE TIME that this was Jaxx and my restaurant. Bayfront is where Jaxx took me on our first date. It is a well-known restaurant, a go-to, white-tablecloth, several-different-types-of-forks place to get a filet on the water, restaurant.

I drag myself into the restaurant, embarrassed to be seen out with Beau, embarrassed, especially to be at Bayfront with him. I nearly throw up when I recognize the hostess: a girl I'd gone to school with, who, not joking, had a crush on Jaxx.

Beau refused to go somewhere else, so I refuse to order anything. Instead, I get straight to the point. I explain all of the things that are truly awful. I tell him that it is not working, and I use the phrase: "no hard feelings" more than once.

As I am getting into it, really diving into the nitty-gritty of the "I don't want to be with you…EVER" speech, Beau pulls out a black velvet ring box from his coat pocket.

"That sucks," Beau says, "because I was going to give you this." His hand shakes as he places the box on the tablecloth between us. "Here, Open it. I want to marry you."

I scoot my chair out from under the table, which is directly under the almost setting sun and leave the restaurant.

"I need to go outside," I say.

"We are outside," Beau says.

Ignoring his dumb remark, I turn around and walk back through the dark, ambient-rich atmosphere that haunts me like an entire crowd of people are laughing at me. My inner voice is talking so loudly I can't shut it out. It's begging me to answer some questions:

How the hell did I get here and how the fuck do I get out before anyone notices where I've been for the past six months? Can we invent time travel? Or a time eraser, like the magic eraser for time rather than walls, or just pretend none of this ever happened. All I wanted to do was to stop drinking. That's it!

The Serenity Journal: No Memories, No Cry

June 29th, 2010:

    I am honestly too afraid of feeling to recount what has happened lately. I will soon though. I have to. I honestly do not think I kept any memories further back then January 6, the day I met the guy who put these diamonds on my finger.
XO Kali Rae

A List of Names

What's backwards about the journal entry on the previous page is that Beau was the cause of so much pain and doubt within me. He was supplying me. He plucked me out of an AA meeting and scooped me up like he was the ask-all guy from Alcoholics Anonymous (AA). The night we met he asked if I would go to the six a.m. meeting the next morning with him. I was up all night organizing. The next morning he talked to me throughout the entire meeting. The next page has an entry that has solely a list of names:

Jaxx, Aaron, Dane, Jason, Jaxx, Aaron, Jaxx, Beau.
Below that is a line and below the line reads:
Check calendars. Check journals, emails too.

June 30, 2010

Beau is still gone and there are so many emotions swimming around inside me. I wish I was happy or at least excited about the prospect of it all. However, I am not ready to commit in that way at all. I am so young!!

Telling Morgan this morning about Beau's proposal, I was almost ashamed and reminded her multiple times that it was a promise ring. I do not want completely drop him like a hot potato because, honestly, Beau is charming when sober. He just needs to lose weight/go to the gym/get his life together/get a job/be making good money as a doctor/act normal/act his age not his shoe size.

I feel like he left the moment he decided to fall off the wagon. That's when he became a lot less than anything close to someone I would look up to.

So now I find out that Jaxx is probably in jail. Haven't been able to get a hold of him, and his friends have no idea where he is either. I just feel a momentary glimpse of excitement surge through my veins thinking of the possibility that I will be going to USC tonight. Blaise is going to be there. It's not that I'm into Blaise but I kind of like the idea of showing myself and everyone that I am not dead. Dead = held down, engaged. I am NOT!!! I also am feeling extreme cold feet towards the whole situation.

Because it's crucial, I've decided to let go of a little bit of my self-consciousness.

Timeline since my move to Los Angeles August 27, 2010:
Aaron Bonaventura
- Sold me first apartment in Los Angeles.
- Wore Crest white strips while showing the apartment; Dad found it odd.
- Wanted me to Facebook him.
- I did on the ride home from LA and we talked online even though Jaxx was mad about it.
- The first night Jaxx was gone, Aaron raped me.
- I felt like there was so much more out there when I met Aaron.
- Picked me up on first date, took me to his house, went in Jacuzzi, blacked out, woke up with hurt ankle. He gave me clothes.
- Promised he was into me.
- I even brought him to Thanksgiving here in Newport, thinking I could fix everything, wanting to have everything not be the way

that it truly was. He had nowhere to go.

Dane
- Met him first day when he brought over his hookah. Jaxx was there too.
- Texted me late at night when I left his apartment: *I can't believe you didn't suck my dick.*
- So drunk I didn't remember anything that happened that night.
- Waited up for him…drinking in the bathroom, alone.
- Hid from him in a bush when I saw him outside the apartment.
- He picked my roommates up from the restaurant underneath the apartment building and never even called me.
- Loved the smell of his place.
- It was another escape.
- During the crazy party at my apartment a few days after I moved in, he rescued me…or I thought he was rescuing me. One wink and I followed him back to his apartment and away from the madness inside mine.

Jason Murray
- How'd we meet?
- Busy, busy boy.
- Became personal trainer.
- Started being verbally abusive, though I didn't notice it as abuse.
- Started being physically abusive, assaulting me. Again, I didn't notice it as abuse.
- Held me at gunpoint and raped me.

Jaxx Moreau (back together in November-ish)
- Jaxx stayed in my apartment the first weekend that I moved in.
- First night back at my apartment after I made appt. with Chai, Jaxx came over and I told him to leave.
- The first night he was gone, Aaron raped me.
- He picked me up from my Aunt's and gave me Percocet for my headache, then he drove me to Teddy's, a popular nightclub, and told me that my awkward sandal-boots were totally nice enough to go inside the nightclub. (See Appendix W.)
- I LOVED the feeling of being with him, so familiar, so in love I couldn't breathe. He was my safety net after having no one on my team for a while.
- We talked about how we would never find someone better, on the bed of his new apartment with our mutual friend, Alexa, in LA.
- I cried tears of joy.
- Started living with him in Los Angeles, instead of my aunt's

house, where I moved in November after my roommates began terrorizing me—literally: One of them slammed my head in a door and screamed at me. The other two were just mean girls, gossipy, making up rumors, getting Dane to turn on me.
- How did I find out he was using again?? Watched the red cap fall to the floor at his apartment.
- January 1, 2010: W/Jaxx at clubs, overdosed on Xanax, Somas and 80's, thought I was going to die. (See Appendices X, W, B.)

Beau Daus
- Met him at AA literally five days after above incident with Jaxx.
- Second date was early morning Alcoholics Anonymous meeting at Lighthouse, then he gave me designer shoes in a juice place parking lot.
- Two weeks after meeting I went to his dad's beach house.
- Proposed to me at Bayfront Restaurant (Jaxx and my favorite spot) the night I was trying to break up with him.
- Got kicked out of my house for stealing my meds.
- Stole money from the woman who hit my car by asking for her to pay the deductible and address the check to him. My dad figured this out later on, when he never received a check for the deductible.
- Got on one knee in movie theater during *Get Him To The Greek* after the restaurant.
- I did not want it, was sick with MRSA.
- OMG the fun we had on Subutec.
- Didn't like the way he looked in his construction clothes.
- I got sick (kidney issues lingering from Topamax) waiting at the fire station, where he was applying to work.

Sitting as close to the door as possible, probably only three to four seats in. I must get back to meetings call these sponsors.

XO Kali Rae

July 1, 2010

I am very nervous about my gum surgery. They screwed up last time and I woke up while they were doing it, and then they gave me so many drugs that I didn't wake up correctly. So, yeah, of course I am a little nervous. Sadly I am more nervous about how I will look after because I have dog training with Stella that night and my neighbor and high school classmate, Elliot, is training his golden retriever puppy in the same class.

12:53 p.m.

I get random surges of depression. This time it was caused by the spellbinding music from the "Twilight" movies. The second book makes so much sense to me that it's hard to read.

8:30 p.m.

I am hoping I get over this depression with a good night's sleep. I hope things turn around while I'm sleeping because I don't know how I am going to make it with this mindset. I feel just so, so alone. And I have an intense feeling of longing and anticipation toward something unknown. Why are nights so lonely? I feel as if the dimming of the night sky brings with it such distraught feelings. Nothing and no one can make me smile. I hope this Seroquel drowns out these destructive thoughts. (See Appendix F.)

XO Kali Rae

July 2, 2010

I am struggling a lot right now and it's hard to even define right from wrong. I know I just need to continue believing that everything will work out in time. I will not be dependent on anyone and I will comprehend the word serenity.

XO Kali Rae

Those Eyes

Look at me.
Those eyes I despise.
I'd cut you deeper
If you'd finally scream.
Tried to steal my dignity.
Your attempt
I shoved back in your face.
Drop your weapon.
You're sick.
Bummer, I'm sicker.
I'll cut up your weapon,
throw it back at you.
You're the reason I made it here.
Tried to slow me down,
hold me back,
and I laugh.
Your tears feed me like
dope
to a dope fiend.
I love it.
Cry harder
until your body feels weak.
Collapse into pitiful remorse,
dumb fuck.
Let's see you try that move again.

July 6, 2010

Day 1

My relationship with Beau will be fine. I will be in easy, fun classes. I will remain sober. Tomorrow will be fun. I will excel at my job. An agency will pick me up quickly. I will have a relaxing, sober summer. My professors will be awesome. My housing situation will be perfect. I will be self-sufficient, yet have a surplus of friends in the program. I will succeed. Stella will be perfectly trained. The program will take away my suffering and bring me that much closer to God I will have an awesome time with Lori one day at a time, one moment at a time.

XO Kali Rae

July 7, 2010

Day 2

Going to my sponsor's house in a little later

So I'm going to another meeting tonight at 7:30p.m. I've been struggling a lot due to the fact that I've been busy since six o'clock this morning. I was called in to work on my day off and just felt awful all day. I really want to take some more Xanax but I know I shouldn't because it will simply make me more depressed.

Later

I'm meeting Beau at 9:30. I'm told to stay away from relationships for a year but for some reason it just makes me a hell of a lot more distraught about staying sober. I am going to live day by day, moment by moment and not screw up my mind any more than it is.

XO Kali Rae

July 8, 2010

Tomorrow will be a new day
I will be happy
I will enjoy tomorrow
I will feel great tomorrow
It will be okay
Write
Paint
Draw
Sing
Guitar
Piano
XO Kali Rae

July 10, 2010

I need to learn how to live in the moment. It will be alright. Tomorrow is a brand new day.
XO Kali Rae

Enough: July 15, 2010

Today is a new day
but I've heard enough
Looked around at a circle
that reminds me I'm alone
not home
the coffee is a couple degrees too hot
And the tiles on the ceiling
I've counted too many times to bring my mind from your steel iron grasp
Yeah, so the past is the past
Stay present today
But today is one of those "all I can do is pray"
I wake up and see your emotionless face
Dream of hurting you so bad
It's not your legs I'd break
For those you can cast and heal
I want to make
That therapy will never be able to heal
I want to break you
Lay down and take it Dirt
I hope the pain never ceases to hinder how you feel
You won't dare to think of another with those slimy, undeserving hands.
Fuck you, you're dead.
I'm driving alone again.
It's become a routine
Drive one direction
U-turn, turn back around
Still not free
The speakers blasting too loud
Can't hear myself think
What a wonderful feeling
Almost tasty as those poppy seeds.
(See Appendix W.)

July 16, 2010

I finally broke it off with Beau, but that doesn't change how hard it is to find out your ex-boyfriend was a compulsive liar, thief and sociopath. I never believed he had really done all of the things he had done until now.

Reasons not to be with Beau...

- Stole money from me from car accident.
- No job @ 27.
- Went to detox and still denies using.
- Stories don't add up.
- Goes to Long Beach for meeting and comes back cracked-out.
- Got MRSA (Whatthefuck?) and then gave it to me.
- Wrote Dr. Scott a letter because my mom said Dr. Scott thought he was odd.
- Never helped with Stella.
- Always wanted sex.
- Never took me out.
- Stole my meds.
- Used my house and family.
- Very clingy and possessive.
- Doesn't really want me to succeed.
- Made me feel like I was wrong when all along he knew it was him.

At times I wish I was Bella. She's allowed to feel that emptiness; she can embrace it and move on. And although I feel a need to do the right thing and block you out, why do I have to please others? I'd give so much to hear your voice. But I fear I'll lose more than I'll gain. I feel so exposed. This is worse than physical aggression. As much as I try to hate you I can't help but feel a pain in my chest thinking of the good times we've shared. I wish I could make you hurt like I do.

Life isn't a game. Sometimes snake eyes just don't cut it and you're gone. I dress up, hoping to pull through. Paint my nails in new and exciting shades. Buy new makeup. But this confusion festers. Why did you have to kick me while I was down?

I scrub off the nail polish. It wasn't changing a thing. You stripped me of the real me, broke my legs, watched me cry, watched me fall.

XO Kali Rae

Stolen: July 17, 2010

Came to me at my lowest of lows
Grabbed my arm before I let his hand go.
Led the way when I stood blind
But you walked me further into the dark

Although I despise the things you did
I cannot get them through my head
That those tear-filled ocean eyes
Could deceive my broken smile

Days pass
You've planted yourself in my thoughts
I try to shake it off
Your hazy gaze reappears
Clearer, stronger, harder to blame

No you never laid hands on me
But you emotionally shackled my wrists
Appeared as if you were here to save me
Ended up picking the wrong seed again
You know I wish you were who you said
I yearn for the days you seemed to glow
And all I remember are the good times
I have to write it out or I fear I'll come running back to you.

I cannot even imagine these facts are true
I thought we were meant to be
Two peas in a pod
Look in your eyes I felt I knew
All the world and all its ingredients and the exact degree on its axis it was turning
Let go of you and my soul sinks, fall to the floor

Do you see what you've done
Yes, I know you always loved me
Got on your knees and confessed this
But it was all too late and way too much too quickly
The scar you cut is far too deep
And secretly I still wish you'd show up at my door
So I could recount for you the stitches that really only belong to you

Why don't you try and lace together the stories I had to
Unexplainable
Whisk me away and let the bad times
The lies, fall to the wayside

July 19, 2010

So I had to leave a meeting tonight. This lady would not stop talking about sexual abuse and I already had to hear her same speech two days ago.
XO Kali Rae

Battlefield: July 19, 2010

Everyday is a struggle
Wish I could let myself cry
Wish I was allowed to hurt
Feel so above the hurt of a broken heart
It's like I've been
misused and abused
Too many times to pull through
I fell victim in my own skin
How the hell do I get sober
when my heart has fallen to the floor
What is there to hold on to
I wish I felt that I deserved to live my dreams
OR simply deserved to live
a happy life
I fear my entire life will be an unbelievable battle

Think You In: July 19, 2010

Don't know if I should push you out
Or think you in
My mind is racing again.
It's chasing shadows of memories
But there are so few
I don't get why I wasted my time and energy on you.

July 24, 2010

I definitely should have done this sooner.

The first step...

Powerless over substance, life has become unmanageable. I can't be alone. I haven't felt true joy in years, only euphoria. I cannot connect with others or love anyone. I do not even love myself, for God's sake. Sadly, as I write this the void in my abdomen grows. I'm empty now, no strings to grab, not even threads. I've been torn open, exposed. I don't have a cloying boyfriend to use, nor can I take anything to relieve this constant feeling of inadequacy.

It is day twenty and I know it has to get better, easier in some way or another. I just can't stand the depression, loneliness, speeding through life and forgetting my past. I cannot do this anymore. So here it is:

- rape
- hit
- work
- loved ones
- health
- reliance
- suicidal
- hateful
- so unconfident
- needy (secretly)
- controlled by others
- uneasy
- panicky
- embarrassment

It is extremely hard to start this process, recounting the extremes that have put me in this situation. I can't listen to music without hurting and I haven't picked up my guitar or learned how to play the keyboard I was given by my grandmother.

I cannot have healthy relationships. I don't want anyone to need me and I do not want to need anyone. I want to live in a cave and disconnect from this impossible world. While with Jaxx life was great, or so I think now that I look back on it. However, I cannot keep burying my past.

Even if it kills me to bring it back up, somehow this will work. I will vomit up the bad and bring in a new world and be conscious each day. I've never been lower. Even though it looks like I've got it all. I lost myself so many years ago and I often feel as if my mental and emotional issues are always ready to cut me down when I finally begin to find an inch of steady ground.

I'm always alone, even in a sea of familiar faces. It keeps me busy and my head at bay, which is good, until I'm alone. I do not even know if I am strong enough to write this. I refuse to let myself cry but the quote below struck me deeply:

"*Do not let your hearts be troubled. Trust in God, also in me.*"[3]

I am extremely suicidal right now and I don't know what to do. I honestly do not care about admitting defeat. All I want is to be happy, healthy, centered and successful. Page. 21 of *The Big Book* reads, "Until he so humbles himself, his sobriety—if any—will be precarious. Of real happiness he will find none at all" (W., 1939).

I also highlighted the words "liberation and strength" I cannot wait for that feeling. I cannot even imagine the thought of serenity. When I imagine serenity, I think of Norcos crushed up and shaken in a bottle of water, oxy until I cannot feel a thing, drinking until my mind shuts off, as many Xanaxs as it takes to forget and enough Adderall to keep from sleeping. Cocaine is even better because it provides both the happiness and energy—like a manic state in which you can do it all. I am fucking powerless over substances and chemicals that alter my mind. I would do anything to get out of my head.

Even when I'm high I have to blast music to get the thoughts to simmer down and keep the TV on meaningless reality shows. I do anything to silence my head. I have such a long list of things I want to do but haven't accomplished. And just thinking about the time I've lost and continue to lose actually makes me want to use so much more.

Can't I just at least have a pulled-together, sexy man to help me through this grieving process? I guess that's another unmanageable, unhealthy addiction. I cannot wait until I can wake up in the morning and feel as if I can live each day moment by moment enjoying the process—not continually waiting or regretting or feeling as if I lose more and more time as the day progresses.

"Our admissions of personal powerlessness finally turn out to be firm bedrock upon which happy and purposeful lives may be built."[4]

Geez, I just took a walk with Stella, Elliot, and his new golden retriever puppy and he truly makes me happy. I'm not saying we should date but I LOVE being around him. It is so difficult for me to deal with people, I feel so awkward and I always feel like everyone is judging me. I am a LOVE

---

[3] John: 14:1, New American Standard Bible.
[4] *The Big Book of Alcoholics Anonymous*

addict. However, I abhor sex. I am always scared of it. It turns my stomach inside out to think about it. No wonder I have to get fucked up into oblivion to have sex or show anyone any kind of affection. Using got me beaten, used, raped and raped at gunpoint while under the influence. The worst part of that was the fact that I kept running back into their arms. I was addicted to feeling. I was addicted to these sick, sick relationships.

XO Kali Rae

July 30, 2010

Wow! Six days it's been because I cannot build the confidence to write. I beat myself up every day all the time. I feel like I am not sure AA is the place for me. I am prescribed certain medications and when I take them I feel like I shouldn't count that day as a sober day.

Or like if I don't take a run with my dog and hit up the 6:30 a.m. meeting, then I am a failure. I have been working so much I have not been able to write, play guitar, or be with Stella. So here it goes:

When I was using, I lost time.

Memories are basically nonexistent.

The things I cherish the most I could not love because I don't love myself. I have never felt true love for anyone. I used guys like drugs, as numbing devices, anything to get me out of me

I am powerless over so many things that I actually believed I controlled very well.

The feeling that stretches and swells in my stomach is unbearable when I am alone. I cannot manage it. Only substance calms the anxious depression.

The many times I have tried to drink moderately turned out the way one would suspect.

I am still on the meds that I have abused many times in the past and although I take them, they don't work the same anymore. Instead, I feel like the disease took control of me, even if I don't abuse them.

It's a difficult road to travel.

XO Kali Rae

July 30, 2010

Wow! Six days it's been because I cannot build the confidence to write. I beat myself up every day all the time. I feel like I am not sure AA is the place for me. I am prescribed certain medications and when I take them I feel like I shouldn't count that day as a sober day.

Or like if I don't take a run with my dog and hit up the 6:30 a.m. meeting, then I am a failure. I have been working so much I have not been able to write, play guitar, or be with Stella. So here it goes:

When I was using, I lost time.

Memories are basically nonexistent.

The things I cherish the most I could not love because I don't love myself. I have never felt true love for anyone. I used guys like drugs, as numbing devices, anything to get me out of me

I am powerless over so many things that I actually believed I controlled very well.

The feeling that stretches and swells in my stomach is unbearable when I am alone. I cannot manage it. Only substance calms the anxious depression.

The many times I have tried to drink moderately turned out the way one would suspect.

I am still on the meds that I have abused many times in the past and although I take them, they don't work the same anymore. Instead, I feel like the disease took control of me, even if I don't abuse them.

It's a difficult road to travel.

XO Kali Rae

July 31, 2010

The first step is taking incredibly long because I feel the need to paint a portrait instead of draw a sketch. I have never been so afraid to actually look in the mirror and pull out all of the things I've stuffed way down inside. When I shine the flashlight down this endless abyss, I feel that the dim light will never be bright or strong enough to reveal what's down there and what is left of the real me. I'm gonna take a shot and begin. I'll try once again to be completely honest with myself . What really is down there?

- Abuse
- Sexual abuse
- Defeat
- Depression
- Mania
- Desperation
- Solitude
- Void
- Pain
- Embarrassment
- Shame
- Confusion
- Lost years
- Unsuccessful attempts
- Boredom
- Endless
- Never-changing
- Lack of self-esteem
- Lack of a clear picture of me
- Broken dreams
- Lies
- Broken hearts
- Loss
- Loss
- Loss

The clock continues to click away, whether I'm there or not. I often wish I had kept a journal every day over the past nineteen years so that I could remember the good times spent with good people but even more to record the painful "I should have learned from the last time this happened." I can't even believe that my mind has been severely chemically altered for the past six years of my life, probably even longer.

XO Kali Rae

I Don't Wanna Remember: July 31, 2010

If I shine a flashlight
down the dark hallway
of this endless abyss,
I feel the light
will never be bright enough
to reveal what is left
at the end of the madness
at the beginning of the real me.
I don't wanna remember.
I don't wanna forget.
I don't wanna remember.
I don't wanna forget.

I Left: July 31, 2010

Our love was so fake
I toss and turn
laugh and weep

I'm reminiscing,
reaching back to grasp
the days we smiled,
you smiled,
I left.

When I think of love,
I think of drugs.
I said I loved you.
I apologize.
That wasn't me.
I wasn't me.

July 31, 2010

I'm a little bit lost,
and I'm a little bit found.
I appreciate you stealing
the last piece of my plastic crown.
I appreciate you
pulling the thread,
to unravel so elegantly,
all at once,
everything that I'd been trying to hold together.

I'm a little bit lost.
I'm a little bit found.
Look down at my hand,
but all I see is cold ground.
You said you'd always be true,
and I can't argue that.
My picture of you was Picasso and flat.

I'm a little bit lost.
I'm a little bit found.
Still wonder why I seem to want you around.
Feel like another chunk of me was taken
by a loser who had the courage to break me.
And I stare in the mirror.
I look myself up and down.
Still an ocean away
from loving the smile on my face.
And I wish I could laugh
even more I could cry,
jealous of tears shed by those
who aren't lost in the storm.
Heard a song the other day.
It told me what I already knew.
I'm fighting insecurities,
stirred up in my own head, a homebrew,
and I think to myself,
if they only knew.

August 1, 2010

I just left a speaker meeting because I didn't feel like it was helping anything. I really wanna use and now I feel super guilty, but I want Aiden [guy from AA] to love me. I want him to be my first honest relationship. But I know he won't because I don't know him and now I leave for Los Angeles to open the store.

When I use I am codependent on everyone and everything around me. I cannot try and push these feelings any deeper. There is a void of darkness in my gut. I hate nighttime. All I want is an escape from the pain.

- Lies, lies, lies
- Unattainable expectations
- Unfinished projects
- Chaos
- Loss of personal connection
- Running into the arms of abuse
- Unable to help the obsessive thoughts

No drugs will ease the pain anymore. I am overwhelmed with everything. I've lost my dignity, my innocence, my soul, my passions, my patience, my trust in anyone, the ability to relate to and enjoy others. I can't stand to be alone and I wish I could take it all back, but I can't and I'm embarrassed, lost and a true addict of all trades.

XO Kali Rae

Returning the Ring[5]

Drove all the way there,
just to drive myself home.
Put the car in park,
then the moonlight changed its tone.

Drove over the hill,
rubber burned the cement,
foot firm on the gas,
I was ready to repent.
Drove over the hill,
heart turned to stone,
tumbling the ring between my young fingers,
removing it promptly,
from its center-console home.

But the parking space felt
just a tad bit too small.
Just a tad bit too small.
Just a tad bit too small.
And my cheeks all the while,
like a porcelain doll

Put the car back in drive.
I'm too far from home.
I'm too far from home.
I'm too far from home.
I drove all the way here,
just to drive home alone.

---

[5] written two months later

2 Back to the City, Classes in the Hills

The adventures of a young girl moving from Newport Coast—a luxurious beach town—to a much bigger bubble, but a bubble nonetheless, the city of Los Angeles. (Blog Description, August 2011)

Not a Fashion Virgin

In high school, I got a gig with a fashion designer/stylist in Hollywood. It was magical. I had discovered this whole new world, a world that only I could uncover because I had the balls to walk into a million fashion houses with a resume. I ended up in the perfect spot: hand-gluing rhinestones to the back of the tights of an *American Idol* performer in the very center of Hollywood.

I got to learn about the culture of cross-dressing, by being exposed to Marcus and his fabulously kind fiancé, Hunter, who always made me feel not only welcome but necessary. He made me feel like I was integral to the group. Marcus introduced me to everyone who entered the studio, including all of the artists' managers, and spent most of the day sewing or putting together new pieces, chatting with me about this and that and showing me everything from how to properly sew on a button, to how to correctly organize a megastar's closet.

I got to see the fabric room and learn about how he came up in the industry. The studio space doubled as a mini-shop and event space, had a mirrored room for hair and makeup and ample space to do the actual photoshoots. This same area was utilized for the weekly yoga class on Sunday. The patio shared a wall with a very popular club in Hollywood at the time, and I truly felt in the know.

Marcus's place was lined with x-rated paintings of male genitalia, and the studio was full of interesting designs for men's strap-ons and different kinds of underwear. It was all tasteful, of course, but it also made me feel like I was not a fashion virgin. I'd seen it all, I thought, and nothing fazed me.

On top of being assistant to the head designer and stylist, Marcus, I also served as resident mannequin whenever Marcus needed something fitted for an artist.

"Arms up!" he said, and I stripped down in the name of fashion!

At times I felt uncomfortable, but it was more while staring at some of his paintings. I thought I was well seasoned when it came to weird jobs and adjusting quickly to unusual situations, especially after working for Marcus.

All of this is to say, when the photographer at my new job with RucKus presented himself as a nice guy, I had nothing to measure that against in a negative way. My job with RucKus had recently turned into a corporate internship. I felt more confident than ever. So when Cameron, the photographer for the company, asked me to model for him, my answer was a thrilled "Yes!"

I was flattered. Cameron had quite the following for his mega-hipster—I'm talking lives in Venice and rides a bike to work—blog. He is a critical part of the cutting-edge company, the design, and marketing of it, at least.

A Corporate Fashion Internship

I am well aware that the store focuses most of its attention on an image, and that Bentley appreciates my body the same way Marcus did.

Bentley often comes into the store with new designs and asks for me by name. He drapes his newest creation over me, often pinning the top to accommodate my less than adequate chest area or tighten the waist so that my butt isn't drowning in fabric. It is interesting to listen to the men's critiques as Bentley steps back to look at me like a mannequin, commenting, no holds barred about the way it does or does not showcase my figure.

"It falls oddly on her. Look at the bust," Bentley says as he flags Joaquin over.

"Yeah, it's a lot of fabric around the butt," Joaquin says.

"Yeah…she is tiny, though," looking up from his default stance: one arm like a seatbelt across his body, acting as a fulcrum to rest the other elbow on, which holds his chin up.

When Bentley is thinking about a possibility, he outstretches his "chin-rest" arm, tilts his head to the right and shifts his weight before coming over to re-pin or undress me a little.

I like studying the tattoos on his hands as he goes through the motions.

Bentley and Joaquin (the head of merchandising and marketing) aren't ever really looking at me.

I have the freedom to pretty much look where I want. That part is fun. I am like the Mona Lisa; the piece of art that looks back.

"You are super hot," Bentley says nonchalantly.

He walks toward me, pulling a few safety pins out of his pocket. He positions his body centimeters away from mine as he reaches through the halter top to pull together the fabric between my breasts, the place where there should be cleavage.

Getting a little touchy huh?" he whispers to me and then asks Joaquin, "How's this?"

"Try from behind," Joaquin says.

Bentley widens his stance and drives his hand down the back of the jumper.

Having obeyed the instructions to go commando (so as not to "ruin the line") I jump as he slides his cold hand down my body. He "follows the line" of the jumper all the way around my hips and pulls the fabric tighter around my hips. He stands directly behind me. I can smell cigarettes on his breath and his cologne is strong, but it smells good. His moto leather jacket adds to the equation.

"You look beautiful, Kali," Bentley whispers before popping his head out from behind to ask Joaquin, "How about now? Good?"

"Yeah. way better. Kali, you cold?" Joaquin asks in his thick Parisian accent. He laughs as he pulls a lighter from his front pocket and lights the cigarette hanging from his mouth.

"Don't listen to him. He's a jerk. You can keep the jumper, Kali. I love it on you. Please wear it for the opening tonight," Bentley says.

"Okay! Thank you so much!" I reply.

"I want you there in my jumper, with stilettos, black and red lipstick…oh my God…YES, a top-hat. Definitely need to get you a top-hat to try…" Bentley continues as he walks around the concrete showroom space.

"Just Kali?" Joaquin asks accusingly.

Joaquin's the guy who brought me from the storefront in Newport Coast up to the corporate offices in Los Angeles. I planned for it, though. When I heard that corporate was coming in, I made sure to find out who, what, when and where, as well as purchase a new RucKus shirt/dress that would work with boots and a belt: I do my homework.

I was working alone that day. And after eagerly helping Joaquin re-merchandise the space of the white-walled, concrete–floored, all-windows shop, I got a chance to speak about my experience with fashion and ask for an internship with him at the corporate office.

"Did you go to FIDM?" Joaquin asks. His Parisian accent matches his mostly gray, wolf-like hair. I'm not sure if his hair is dyed or if that's a natural color.

"No," I say.

"I can't take you," Joaquin says looking back down at his phone.

"I'm a UCLA student, and I worked directly for Marcus Morello. I will work my ass off for you," I say to the top of Joaquin's wolf-colored head.

Joaquin looks back up quizzically, "Okay, how about you start tomorrow…in LA."

"I work tomorrow in this store. Should I switch my shift…or—" I think out loud.

"You want the job or no?" Joaquin retorts.

"Yeah, I just—should I find someone to cover my shift?" I ask in a daze from the impromptu offer.

"What?" He is staring at his phone now, uninterested. "Yeah, do whatever you need to do, just be downtown tomorrow. I've got to run. Love that dress on you."

He snaps a photo without warning as he leaves the store.

"Ciao!" he shouts from the purple backdrop of the outdoor mall's evening sky.

The owner of RucKus, Bentley, grabbed prime real estate in August of 2010, snatching up a third location in a brand new mall on the coast of Los Angeles. I have only been working at corporate for a few weeks, but Bentley wants his favorite sales girls to open the new store for him, wearing mandatory stiletto heels and black top-hats and, of course, and one of his personally designed garments. Cameron and I haven't crossed paths yet at the corporate office. I will meet the photographer at the opening of the new store in Los Angeles.

The Photog

"So I hear you're a writer?" says a voice to the left of me.
The sound of a camera clicks, and I look up from the clothing rack I'm organizing in stilettos and a top-hat. I look toward him in an awkward position. The sounds quickens: Click…click.click.click. click.click.click.click…Click.

"Stop!" I laugh. "Yeah, I write. How did you know?"

The furious sound of more camera flashes allows me to understand that he doesn't care to hear my answer.

"Wait, do that look again," Cameron says.

"What look?" I ask, genuinely confused.

"Bend over and pick that up again," Cameron says.

I drop the canvas tag on the brushed concrete showroom floor again and skillfully, using my dance background, do a bit of a bend-and-snap motion. I twist his way, flashing a very cute duck face at the end.

I hate posed photographs. And this is not an exception.

Cameron drops the camera by his side.

"I got a good one anyway," he says and picks the camera up again. "Why don't you like to take photos?" Cameron asks. His eyes are stuck in the viewing lens, mouth scrunched on one side, the sound of the shutter click is nonstop. He moves around in a sort of way that makes the conversation casual, yet he's capturing the perfect angles while doing so. "You're beautiful; why don't you model? You could model and make a ton of money."

He's distant as he snaps away; he is in the zone, reciting, what I guess is the usual script. But I don't expect that comment.

"Well thank you," I say and laugh nervously. Thanks, Mom, for making me blush-proof. "I don't have head shots or anything."

"I can do those for you. Whenever you want, I'm down to shoot those for you, for free, of course," Cameron says.

"Really? That would be like really awesome! Why?" I ask.

He continues to snap away.

"Because I feel like you're a good person. And I'd like to help you. Also, you make for beautiful subject matter. Win-win for me," Cameron replies.

Cameron is a tall, slender, definition of hipster photographer-guy. He has the plain white tee, rolled up a couple of times at the sleeves, the tortoise-shell oversized, circle sunglasses, light-colored pin-rolled Levis that meet his leather, I call them "dad shoes," but they probably have a better name.

This chatter while he snaps photos of me continues throughout the next three opening days of the store. The photographs Cameron takes are some of my very favorite photos of all time. And they are all done without my even noticing. I get a devilish look in my eye when I do notice, and that proceeds to ruin the following frames with a tongue, or a finger, or the pursing of my lips: total rock-star, NOT.

The opening of the store is a blur of getting the space ready, changing in the back to work the floor and smiling in stilettos as the enormous influx of shoppers overtake the cement floors.

"Come out with me tonight. A few of us are going to this thing in Venice. You should cruise," Cameron says.

"I—" I start.

"Just meet me there. I live around the corner. Let me buy you a drink. We'll talk business, your headshots…here," Cameron says. He holds out his phone. "Put your number in and I'll hit you up in an hour or so."

Caught off guard, I type in my number, thinking nothing of the coworker's gesture. I want to hear what he has to tell me about blogging. And I also really want headshots taken. He seems like a normal guy. And his blond hair, parted carefully on one side, and slicked over, reminds me of my hometown. He reminds me of the surfer/hipster boys I grew up around. He is safe.

All Heroin, Not Chic

The photoshoot is fun, random but fun. I am mostly in control, which I don't quite understand because he is the professional.

The outfits are destructive. And, at one point, Cameron has me wash my makeup off so that my mascara runs down my face.

I do so willingly as well as pose atop a mattress in the street without much thought.

Because of what had happened when I was unconscious the night after I met him in Venice, I expect to hang with him after the photoshoot. Or at least, to "Netflix and chill," as kids say these days, aka to be treated like a friend, at least. But when the shoot finishes, and we are walking back to his little house filled with his hipster things, Cameron's demeanor changes.

I watch four women walk up the wood plank steps into the house. The door is left open, like an open art space.

"Thank you, Cameron," I say.

"Yeah, sure. That was fun or whatever," Cameron says. He is staring down at his phone, preoccupied.

I dig a little; things don't seem right, "Are you doing anything tonight?"

"No," Cameron says.

"Okay, I get it. Is she an ex-girlfriend?" I ask, referring to the girl who just entered his home.

"No," Cameron says, detached. He looks up from his phone.

"So last night, I don't remem—" I begin, wanting to get something off of my chest from the night earlier, to clarify what happened when I was unconscious.

He cuts me off. "You were fun; it was funny. Glad you came out."

"Yah, but—" I say and give up as I watch his eyes scan the display of his large Nikon.

As we walk into the small house, the group of thirty-ish women is laughing, all wearing knit sweaters, high-waisted jeans and hats that probably have special names—the big, round hipster ones. A brunette in black looks me up and down.

"Is this your latest, Cameron?" she asks.

She turns to her Bohemian-chic buddies to laugh that mean-girl laugh, the one where you want to either tell them they're worthless or run, suddenly feeling completely worthless yourself.

Waltzing in with smeared mascara, fishnet tights on my arms, and shorts I'd never worn with clunky, very expensive, sheer front, zip-up black stilettos, didn't exactly feel worthy in front of the group wearing effortlessly thrown-together light-colored Levi jeans and white flowy sweaters. I could feel their disdain from the door, and it is growing.

"I'm gonna go change and head out," I say, excusing myself to go to his appropriately decorated terra cotta bathroom.

"Thank you, Kali. I'll let you review the final blog post," Cameron says.

Needless to say, I never got to review the final blog post. The story ends with a blog post that, to put it lightly, makes me look like a drug-addicted whore. He cropped each of the black-and-white photos down to a crotch, or an arm, a side-boob, at one point. Cameron chose the photos where we were playing around with "crazy," when he instructed me to splash water on my face, tousle my hair, and rub my eyes to smear the black eye-makeup.

I just look all heroin, not chic.

August 29, 2010

Mikah: I met him at a party that my cousin took me to after a photoshoot with Cameron that ended badly. At first it went well with Cameron. He even invited me to his home to watch a movie and drink a beer.

XO Kali Rae

Mikah

Mikah wrote me song after song, and he also sang them to me too. So if the question is, "Has anybody ever written anything for you?" I can say yes, multiple things. If he had the confidence, the dude would be famous, no questions asked.

I was fascinated by the pain in his vocals. It spilled out of him. He lured me in with a good attempt at passing off a City and Colour song as his own. And, after a long night of boy band vocal crooning and his ability to make me feel so utterly held-up and hanging on to the lyric, I found myself caught in a contradiction.

Mikah did end up writing songs, I mean actually writing them. And some were even better than that City and Colour song he tried to pull off.

In one song he wrote after a visit, years later, he confesses his undying love and asks me to forgive and forget and to just have fun with him forevermore. He pleads with me while I sit, still torn up by the fact that Mikah could make what we had into some backward romance drama love-song.

The days of my relationship with Mikah are fueled by Jack and Coke and little Russia in West Hollywood, when I should be studying for my Shakespeare 101 class. There is beauty in the destruction of us both. Mikah comes from a background that lends itself well to playing the part of the passive instigator, but I don't see that his tricks are wrapping me up in their charm: presenting themselves as wounds he is still licking from the tragedy.

Mikah introduces me to sad alternative music and the best flea markets on Melrose. He also shows me the side of LA that does care and will take you in off the street. I meet some of my favorite people when I am with Mikah. And I love writing songs in old band t-shirts on the dusty wood floor of his apartment.

Mikah lives with Becca. Becca has overly bleached blonde hair, empty packs of hipster cigarettes strewn around her trendy room and a shawl that is attached to her somehow, in some way, at all times. Her room looks like an old-school Anthropologie ad: Polaroids wall to wall.

I love the chaos because it is organized, young chaos. It is okay to not be okay in that apartment.

Two twin brothers, Seth and Savan, live with Becca most of the time. I can't tell them apart. They are "actor/models" who prefer to book gigs as a pair.

Savan is struggling with a lingering heroin addiction. He recently got sober. I spend one morning taking a very grateful Savan to the methadone clinic.

Becca is in love with Seth, who treats her like shit.

September 6, 2010

I am finally getting the tattoo I've wanted forever.
XO Kali Rae

Poems From a New/the Same Place: Fall 2010

Cold: September 7, 2010

Sometimes I ache so bad,
I feel my blood has gone cold.
I try to smile
but the tears run dry.
And all I know
is it hurts.
Baby, you can't heal this mind.
It's been driven insane far too many times.
By the men who've more than deceived her.
Been treated like dirt.
You'll have to wait for the life to come back,
The warmth left my hands sixteen years ago,
Baby don't make this
Something we both know it's not.

Sometimes I Wish: September 9, 2010

It's true that I sit in the quiet and reminisce.
And it's true that sometimes I wish on a fallen lash
that I'd never locked eyes with you
closed my eyes in a dizzy whirl and seen something
I'll never have the strength to let go of
Yeah sometimes I block out the sound
of your casual cunning words
overwhelming my barriers
you have a tendency to knock them all down
and I don't think you're ready.

Suck It Up: September 9, 2010

Suck it up
Drink it down
Shut your mouth
Boy, hold me down.

Don't ever take my hand,
slip your fingers in between,
I hate the feeling.
It makes me sick,
like champagne
& JD and coke
and memories.

Eye fucked you
till your lashes fell clean.
I apologize that my net has you stuck
Baby struggle till you're dead in
hate for the love I've captured you in.

Let's take a dive,
you go first,
forgot to tell you one thing.
I'm not falling with you
and that pool's not too deep

I'm not an angry person.
Searched long and hard to pull
that emotion
from the dungeon I've locked it in.
Sorry, Baby,
there's nothing left here to see,
It's called
the "I Don't Give a fuck"
gene.

September 10, 2010

I will do so
Fuck it
My wall built itself back stronger.
How can I trust someone else
When I don't even know myself
I'm numb
And I'd rather not pretend to play
Or to be "the way."
I'm an unprecedented mess,
leave me now
Or the sneeze will come from you.

Her Own Space: October 3, 2010

Open the door upon a third-world country.
Foreign as a cat,
swimming in a backyard pool.
The clutter, the mess, the imminent stress…
of cardboard boxes tossed carelessly into corners.
Just another day at work,
for the couple men driving the U-Haul van.
The movers drive away,
She's left alone to become acquainted with her new home.
Please turn on the light.
Voices echo into the night.
"Now you've found a place to call your own"
"No regrets, look you've got your own home!"

Thrown lazily into whatever corner's convenient,
stacks of dusty song lyrics, old furniture,
piles of memories yet to unfold.
Lost as an ant,
running down the wrong hole,
needing a navigation device.
Waiting for the place to ignite,
To fight,
against the slowly falling Sun.

To be replaced,
by the doom-filled Moon;
Dark.

Electricity is absent from the scene.
It will be black tonight.
Bought too many candles to count.
Lying on the itchy, gray, carpeted floor.
Spots on the ceiling make ominous marks,
on the crisp image she held close to my heart.

Dwindling wicks struggle to keep the cave warm.
Clinging to side of the rock-wall,
searching for the piton,
but there's nothing's visible to grab.

Brisk air nipping,
no heat to warm cold fingers,
exposed skin shuttering,
with windows left wide open:
No landlord to fix the broken latch.
They stay open.

Pull me away from the façade of this fireplace.
Let the plumes from the fire bring relief from the mire.
"Ignite!" she says, "Ignite!"

No need for superfluous strife,
"Ignite."

The fireplace is nothing but a warming device,
yelling into the anciently painted walls.
The paint is stripped obnoxiously from the front door,
in places splattered in dry pieces across the lonely floor.

Cobwebs seem the only things alive in this place.
The only living,
breathing organism aside from her mourn-stricken face.

The Effects of Studying for an Exam Given by Professor Divine: Fall 2010

The stagnant air begins to feel like a mallet
Unforgiving migraine fingers wrap my head in a noose
My hands—cold, clammy and uneasy
Rally only to loosely grasp that regal #2 pencil
It is only now that I am horribly regretting the all-nighters.

My eyes sting
They wander
Then shut
But open before the room begins spinning.

The pressure surmounts making me heave
Professor worriedly asks, "Are you alright?!"
"No! The 72 hours of studying was all a waste of time."
My stomach jumps and sways its contents into my mouth
Forcing me to swallow not only my pride
But the horrid contents my body has devised.

Finally nausea overcomes the ability to think
All-nighters regretted
I grit my angry teeth.

For the notes I had typed out so furiously
Left me a void of nonsense mixed heavily by the need to sleep
No hope, no inspiration
Nor the ability to pass the exam
Given in the usual overly generous time span.

The purple circles looked painted under my eyes
So dark they could be recognized by the blind
I'm sick and unable to answer 50 of 60 questions asked
Dreamt up by Professor—let's call him "Divine."

Falling Faster: Fall 2010

Looking down from above the ravine falls drastically
Looking down from above the ravine falls drastically
Climbing up the precipice a walk back in time
I take it step-by-step sullen whiskey on my breath
Never crossed my mind to reconstruct this purposeful death.
Looking up at the clouds I believe I've got it down
My life is a looking glass I'm waiting to be found.
HE's watching from below as I take the final blow.
HE's watching from below as I take the final blow.
Falling like a stone and no the river does not flow.
Looking up from the ravine I feel a tad serene.
Looking up from the ravine I feel a tad serene.
Like addiction is used to describe the relentless fiend.

Galveston Falling Away: Fall 2010

Calm water, smiling faces and fresh fish—
Memories unlacing with each crackling whip.
Falling like Alice down the rabbit hole of watery bliss.
I'll wait below the anger of the storm.
I'll grip fast to the grainy ocean floor.
I take on another wall of water.
Life-saver.
Life-taker.
He looks at me for the last time,
As he struggles to make it ashore.

I Love You, Maybe: Fall 2010

Yearned to hear
them,
Those Three Words,
Yet found no comfort in;
"I love you too Baby Girl."
Those Three Words
So often cast off as cliché.
Perhaps they are more than the reputation they've endured.
Perhaps they could bring the night back today?
Could they lead the guppies back to school?
Organize the V-shaped gull migration?
Over the hump
And mountain
World.

Chains: Fall 2010

That night,
enraged, you said:
"You just don't have what it takes."

I just cracked your ego,
with or without
your drunken approval.

Your exclamations,
taken with a happy pill.
Not the usual grain of salt.

In the space
made treacherous
by your cold-cuts
by your cold, heavy, constraints.

Am I Lost or Was I Left: Fall 2010

The photograph is dull,
yet the meaning all too bright.
Brighter than the dozen balloons,
I hold tight.
I hold tight.
Goodnight.

Grandmamma.
To you, I hold tight.
And Grandpapa,
you are the light.
The tales of the balloons fall,
like your stories, your promises,
that never revealed themselves.
They never came true.
Stories, promises…
they never went nowhere at all.
Broken promises
Leave broken men.
Daddy? Why couldn't you have been,
at least in the auditorium,
to watch me star as the Little Drummer Boy?

Like the strings that strangle,
my four-year-old fingers,
from the inflated promises,
that strangle my four-year-old tears. And I was all but four years,
But I knew up from down,
And I knew I'd been thrown around.

So, Grandmamma.
To you, I hold tight.
And Grandpapa
I still see your light.
So, Grandmamma,
With your flashlight,
and Grandpapa,
with batteries galore,
as I grew older—
just like at age four—

you lit up the night.
When the abyss seemed endless,
my two shining lights,
took me back home.
And I know now,
That I am never really alone.

Fractured Planet: Fall 2010

There is promise that this broken world will heal its fracture,
Pangaea broke apart and much was left by its fracture.

"Soccer" or "Football", which is the correct word for the game?
Americans focus on plays that cause us to fracture.

A migraine pounds until it strikes the back of a sore skull,
Neck bones seem to play musical chairs before they fracture.

Take a shot, ask what I believe in, I'll tell you upfront,
It's a world that stands stronger than Pangaea, no fracture.

Is there a break in the Great Wall of China, I dare ask,
Could've been risky in battle if the wall had a fracture.

Did Apollo 13 gaze upon an undivided globe?
From out there in space, no one would see the looming fracture.

There is a cough at the end of my name, a Pal I am,
Chi is pronounced "key" and spelled Qi, I abhor the fracture.

Your Worst Enemy: Fall 2010

A Black Crow flew over her.
Matched her nail polish,
And left her undecided.

Could've easily been a sign,
Dropped her off on floor thirteen,
Laughed and said goodbye.

But…

Instead she let her mind wander,
And a different path she chose to squander.

Refused, she did—
The relentless, ruthless, ridicule,
That a mind at thought does ponder.

But one cannot refuse the mind,
So, she went with it.
And it went beyond her.

And now she is alone again.

Her thoughts swirl,
Whirl into a gloomy sky of ash,
A plume of nuclear rises from her head.

A mushroom cloud of indecision,
Indecency and in doubt.
Perhaps comparable to the mind of certain presidents,
When placed in heat.

Da Vinci's Muse: Fall 2010

Her eyes reign the perceiver.
She breathes with every expecting glance,
each spectator receiving the response
they so hoped
they would.
Because she could,
reawaken them.
Just for a moment,
just to remind them,
that they should still believe in magic.

And Da Vinci feels no remorse.
No one even knows her true name,
Or the books she liked or the dreams she had
Or even the tragedies that life rolled into her fleeting time here.
And a portrait doesn't say much about countenance.
And they say
"Such fame, perhaps given to an undeserving woman."
But she was…
She was only special after she died.
She was only special after some man made her his experiment.
She was only special after she died.
She was only special
She was only
She was
She
She was not special.
It was her eyes that were special.
It is her eyes,
At least her eyes move.

What to Make of It All: November 25, 2010

Although I feel,
That thinking may steal,
The glory I feel,
As I bask in my own element.
Thinking does too,
Tell me the truth,
And does its best,
To leave me unglued,
Missing you.
All of you.
And that part that I thought was you too.
For as far as I know,
Trees do not grow,
After storms have devoured their roots.
For as far as I know
Trees do not grow
After monsoons have torn them asunder.

Dr. Braun

Walking into the counseling center, I wonder why there isn't a more secretive entrance. The waiting room is the size of a small apartment, with walls separating different sections of it. Chairs are lined up, one right after the other; some rows are back to back, others against windows or walls. It is huge.

I feel for an instant that maybe seeing a psychologist is a private thing. I always make information about my health readily available to anyone who asks, so it is strange that this thought creeps into my head. I stare out the window and watch the soccer players practice. I had no boundaries before, but I am beginning to build some.

I think part of the reason I am so open about everything is because of where I was raised. Having a therapist is commonplace. If you don't have a therapist, specifically Dr. Whittman, you are kind of boring. I am well aware that certain friends are also seeing Dr. Whittman. I know guys who went to him too, including bad boys. I specifically know an older guy, who I snuck out of my house with, also saw Dr. Whittman. And I wondered what Dr. Whittman thought when I went in there to talk over my angst and spilled about another patient of his.

Having a therapist also meant having a psychiatrist, if you were exotic enough. The idea of having doctors working on your state of mental health is very much the norm in Newport Coast. Unless you have serious issues, like having been in jail or the psych ward (depending on the reason) most of us don't hide information. I wear my new bipolar diagnosis like Two Chainz's necklaces. It makes me feel special. It gives me a reason for feeling different.

In Newport we all joked about being young alcoholics. Every weekend we would scout the best house to pre-game. To qualify as a host you need 1) a house so big that there could be a twenty-person pre-game at one end and a serene, trusting pair of parents on the other, 2) a guest house, or 3) the money to pay for a hotel room. The best was when the parents weren't ever around, especially if they lived in a different country/state. In these cases, the beautifully decorated Newport Coast model home was ours to play house in, and along with it, the fully stocked bar, which would never get old. I liked the glasses and the different ways they were kept. If there was a bar, there was always enough crystal-clear glass to serve a football team, and never one speck of dust.

In Newport, the idea of having issues was an edgy detail. Unless you had a serious hospitalization, you were just one of a community of kids with parents who either paid too much attention to their kid and drugged them out of their minds on prescriptions neatly handed to them during their weekly visit, or didn't pay any attention at all to their children. The latter allowed their kids to host the parties, which sometimes made them the "parents" of the group. They had seen too much in their lives to be like the reckless ones.

"Kali?" a tall, thin man with perfectly combed and parted brown hair says as he scans the waiting room. I wake up from my daydream and stand up. He smiles. "How are you, Kali? Good to see you."

We have never met, so I am already made aware of this guy's affectation.

It doesn't get easier. When I tell Dr. Braun about all of the things that are eating away at me, he doesn't say anything. He stays locked in his holier-than-though persona.

At times, he questions why I think things are my fault or he offers me a tissue, but he has no solutions. I always leave his office feeling more vulnerable, misunderstood and completely stripped: void of my safety net. I want to run back into his office and rip up all the stupid notes I know he will type out once I leave. Years later, I find that these notes are even more thorough, judgmental and overall devastating than I had imagined.

Glancing through Dr. Braun's notes, I feel a sinking feeling as I read, "Says been raped 'a bunch of times.'" It is almost immediately after I have this session that I never see him again. I can tell he doesn't understand. And he makes me uncomfortable. The way he looks at me is a bit too interested.

He is too entwined in what I am saying. He likes to listen to me open up to him about the darkest parts of myself, but he offers no solutions.

He makes me feel insanely vulnerable and more fearful of my situation. He will repeat my feelings about situations, or intuition about people to make me feel the weight of them. There isn't support, rather, more questioning. I sense Dr. Braun doesn't believe me, that he doesn't like me. There is something behind his need for details that feels completely irrelevant to the situation at hand. I don't trust him.

Dr. Braun is a detail-oriented man, as his impeccable medical records

DR. BRAUN (PHD, PSYCHOLOGIST): NOVEMBER 2, 2010

MENTAL STATUS
MOOD: normal/euthymic and sad/depressed
AFFECT: congruent with mood and content.
-Appearance, speech rate and volume, psychomotor activity, orientation, rapport, thought process, perceptions, insight, and judgment are all within normal limits.

AREAS NOT WITHIN NORMAL LIMITS:
Speech rate and volume: soft, some scattering

HISTORY OF PRESENTING PROBLEM:
KW stated that she was "really upset today" b/c her professor called a break in class and "yelled" at her for passing out gum in class and for not knowing how to close a window. KW stated that she did not understand why he was angry and just wanted to avoid conflict. Told Professor Y, "I don't mean to disrespect you. I'll leave now if you want."

DEPRESSIVE SYMPTOMS OR SIGNS
- depressed mood
- loss of interest or pleasure in activities
- change in appetite
- fatigue
- low self-esteem
- trouble concentrating
- sleep difficulty

HARM TO SELF OR OTHERS
CURRENT SUICIDAL CONCERNS?: Yes
Suicidal ideation with plan, but no immediate intent
Denied experience of SI today.
Convincingly endorsed willingness to notify undersigned if SI re-appeared/increased. Stated that SI has been present for "several years." Spoke in future oriented terms regarding job and academics. Emphatically denied intent and stated that she was not feeling suicidal today. Will contact this writer or ProtoCall Hotline if distress levels increase. Also noted that she attends 12 step meetings on a daily basis.
PRIOR SUICIDAL CONCERNS: Yes
SUICIDAL ATTEMPT: During sophomore year in HS - 800 mg of Seroquel
GAF 53

DR. BRAUN: NOVEMBER 5, 2010

MENTAL STATUS
MOOD: normal/euthymic and sad/depressed
AFFECT: congruent with mood and content
-Appearance, speech rate and volume, psychomotor activity, orientation, rapport, thought process, perceptions, insight, and judgment are all within normal limits.

HARM TO SELF OR OTHERS
CURRENT SUICIDAL CONCERNS?: No
No SI today. Stated that she is "responsible" about seeking support (e.g., use of the hospital). Continues to endorse a willingness to contact this writer if SI concerns appear. Will also utilize walk-ins or the ProtoCall Hotline if needed.

TREATMENT NOTES
KW arrived in an overtly stable affective state. Noted that this week she experienced panic episodes about being served a subpoena. Tried to describe the significance of the latter in the context of her life. Agreed to provide a timeline of her life experiences before processing her anxiety. Also agreed to provide RO I's for this writer to speak with her psychiatrist.
GAF: 53

DR. BRAUN: NOVEMBER 15, 2010
Mode of Contact: Telephone

VM left on KR's cell phone answering service proposing dates and times to meet for a follow-up session this week. Call back requested.

DR. BRAUN: NOVEMBER 16, 2010
Mode of Contact: Email
FROM: BRAUN, ALEC J.
TO: WHEELER, KALI RAE

Hi Kali

I hope things are well with you.

I left you a voicemail message yesterday and thought I would follow-up with an email regarding our previous meeting. First of all, thank you for filling out the Release of Information forms. I was successfully able to consult with both parties. Having done so, I secondarily wanted to reschedule a meeting with you this week in advance of our appointment on 11.22 .10. Depending on your availability, we can alternatively schedule a telephone check-in if that would be helpful. So when you have free moment, please feel free to let me know which days and times you are available this week.

On a final note, it may be helpful to recall that CAPS offers walk-in appointments M - F between 10am and 5pm. We also have a ProtoCall Hotline Service xxx-xxx-xxxx which is available 24 hours on weekends and holidays. ProtoCall can also be contacted on M - F from 5pm to 8am. In case of emergency please dial 911 or go to the nearest hospital emergency room.

I look forward to speaking with you soon.

Best wishes,

Dr. Alec Braun.

DR. FIASCHETTI: NOVEMBER 17, 2010
Provigil 200mg. (See Appendix U.)

DR. BRAUN: NOVEMBER 17, 2010
Mode of Contact: Telephone

VM left regarding opening for appointment tomorrow. 11.17.10. Call back requested.

DR. BRAUN: NOVEMBER 22, 2010

MENTAL STATUS
MOOD: normal/euthymic and sad/depressed
AFFECT: congruent with mood and content
-Appearance, speech rate and volume, psychomotor activity, orientation, rapport, thought process, perceptions, insight, and judgment are all within normal limits.

TREATMENT NOTES
KW arrived in an overtly stable affective state. Addressed concerns about mixed support from bf and family regarding medication, medical problems (e.g., dramatic), and requests for help (e.g., crisis). Became tearful as she noted difficulties remembering prior sexual violations. Was able to respond to reflective interventions in order to clarify multiple confounding factors (drugs, ETOH "allergy", manic episodes, stress/anxiety). KW was also able to consider alternative perspectives regarding her self-blame pertaining to prior sexual violations. Safety practices were addressed in order to reduce her stress/anxiety (e.g., with professor who reportedly focuses on sexualized interpretations of poetry) which may trigger anxiety and bipolar episodes. Will meet again tomorrow if KW's schedule permits. Hold was placed.
GAF: 55

DISPOSITION/TREATMENT PLAN
Continue to assess safety; id triggers for bipolar and sexual assault trauma reactions. Stabilize and prepare for referral to BHI. Interval until next appointment: Tentative f/u tomorrow

DR. BRAUN: NOVEMBER 24, 2010
Mode of Contact: Email
FROM: BRAUN, ALEC J.
TO: WHEELER, KALI RAE
SUBJECT: YESTERDAY'S APPOINTMENT

Hi Kali,

I hope things are well with you.

I noticed that you were not able to make it to the appointment I held for you yesterday. When you have time today, or as soon as possible, would you please call me (or the front desk if I am not available) at the telephone number below and reschedule.

Best wishes,

Alec

DR. BRAUN: NOVEMBER 30, 2010

Mode of Contact: Email
FROM: BRAUN, ALEC J.
TO: WHEELER, KALI RAE
SUBJECT: RE: RE YESTERDAY'S APPOINTMENT

Hi Kali,

Thanks for getting back in touch with me. It is indeed a busy time of the school year. I will look forward to meeting with you next week. Please be aware that openings for next week are filling up. As of this morning, there are more openings on Friday.

Best wishes,
Alec

-----Original Message-----
FROM: KALI RAE WHEELER
SENT: TUESDAY, NOVEMBER 30, 2010 9:36 AM
TO: BRAUN, ALEC
SUBJECT: RE: YESTERDAY'S APPOINTMENT

I apologize. I have been extremely swamped with school and finals and everything. I will make an appointment next week.

I am just overloaded with work right now.

Thank you! And I apologize again.

Best,
Kali Rae Wheeler

DR. BRAUN: DECEMBER 6, 2010
Mode of Contact: Email
FROM: BRAUN, ALEC J.
TO: WHEELER, KALI RAE

Hi Kali,

I hope this email finds you making progress with your high workload. With respect to scheduling, I have some openings on Friday (12/10) at 8, 9, or 10am. For the purposes of supporting your self-care, safety, and well-being let's try and meet at one of the above times. Please feel free to email me, or call me at the telephone number below in order to schedule. If these times do not work for you, please also let me know what days and times you are available so that I can keep an eye out for additional openings. Thanks!

Best wishes,

Alec

Truck Driver, December 19, 2010

I'm like a truck driver
Drunk behind the wheel
Driving to a place
That I know
Is not the place
That I should go.

DR. BRAUN: DECEMBER 22, 2010 (EMAIL)
Mode of Contact: Email
FROM: BRAUN, ALEC J.
TO: WHEELER, KALI RAE

Hi Kali,

I hope your winter break is going well thus far.

Since it has been some time since our last appointment on 11.22.10 and you were unable to come in and meet with me since then, I wanted to remind you that we will be closing down for the winter break beginning today at 5pm. I might suggest that you schedule a meeting with Dr. Fiaschetti as needed during our closure.

Also, please recall that we will continue to make the Hotline Service (xxx-xxx-xxxx) available during the entire winter break, 24 hours a day. In case of an emergency please dial 911 or go to the nearest hospital emergency room.

Happy holidays and best wishes,

Alec J. Braun Ph.D.

The Audition

"My audition is in an hour. Can I practice with you?" I ask Mikah.

"Yeah whatever. I really don't think you chose a good joke," Mikah says.

"Okay, well, do you have something better? I have to have a comedy portion. It's mandatory," I say.

"Just not a fucking Kool-Aid joke," he says.

"Okay…well, I'm definitely not doing a Kool-Aid joke," I reply. My nerves are in my throat now. I feel more unprepared than ever. My eyes dart to the clock on the oven. "Shit, Mikah! I have like ten minutes!"

"Relax. Oh, and you sound flat on that Alanis song. Not trying to be picky. Just maybe fix that, like before you sing it. It sounds weird," Mikah says.

"Seriously? How? What??" I ask.

Mikah is a great singer. I inquire further as Mikah unpacks the white, paper bag containing his daily dose of weed. He reaches for a piece of the pizza he ordered for himself.

"You're just off," Mikah says. He takes a bite.

My gaze is fixed. He finally bites the cheese swinging off his piece of pizza.

"How can you even dance with your knee?" Mikah asks.

"What?" I say, pissed.

"Don't be mad. I'm just saying. You know?" Mikah continues chomping.

Gross.

"Kali. Stop...Kali? Okay fine. Don't answer me. But stop looking at me like that," he says.

I look up from the script I've been clenching in my right hand. It's served as a blank staring template for the past few minutes of Mikah's fun little talk.

"I have to go," I say as I grab my bag and leave my apartment, shutting the door behind me.

The Fish Tank Incident

Mikah laughs condescendingly as he bounds across the studio apartment into the kitchen.

"Oh, you think this fish tank is yours?" Mikah taunts.

I study his movements cautiously.

"What are you doing?" I ask. I stumble over my words and then continue, "Yes, duh, it's mine. I paid for it. You made me pay for it! I've spent a thousand dollars on that fish tank! And tell me again why I would want a thirty-gallon fish tank in my first apartment?"

Mikah is searching under my sink for something. "I bought every one of those fish. They belong to me," Mikah says.

"You have got to be kidding me. I have receipts. Good luck proving that, Mikah," I say.

"You have not done one thing to take care of these fish. Name one thing you've done. Actually, don't. I do everything; I'm taking them," Mikah says. Mikah's aggression is building steadily.

"You are not taking one thing from this apartment!" I shout.

"Try and stop me," Mikah says.

"I'm calling my dad. I'll take you to court. I paid over twenty-five hundred dollars for this stupid ass fish tank that I never wanted all because you told me you'd pay me back. You are not taking one more thing from me. You've taken enough," I say.

The last comment hits hard: good. I see it on his face; he finally gets it. He knows what he's done. I pick up the phone to dial my father.

"I'm taking these fish," Mikah passes me, finally making it out of the kitchen. He's holding the green fish net in one hand and has a Ralph's paper bag in the other.

"Dad! Mikah is being insane… No… Yes… YES… He is trying to take the fish and the tanks that I paid for. Whatever! No!… He's just taking it. He told me he'd pay me back, but he never did!" I'm shouting into the phone.

He dips the net into the beautiful fish tank we decorated together. Mikah painted the back with glow-in-the-dark paint while I was in class one day. It looks like the actual ocean at night.

Mikah shoves around the neon cave figurine housing the daddy cichlid. He moves it with the thick green wire of the net. The aggressive upheaval of the tank's rocky bottom releases a brown cloud of uneaten fish food and grime into the surrounding water.

Stunned, I drop the phone.

"Mikah! What are you doing?!" I shout.

He slams the biggest Cichlid up against the side of the glass tank, pinning it between the wire of the net and the glass of the front panel of the tank. He's slides it up the glass.

I wince.

It's the green and blue fish: Bruin. He's the father of the twenty-three baby cichlids roaming the tank. He's the size of my fist and a mean sucker, but beautiful nonetheless. He is my favorite, aside from the mini shark-fish I named Meh; the smaller of two received the partner name, Yew.

"Stop! Stop it! Stop!" I shout.

Mikah lifts the fish, in the net, above the water line. With one hand he's pinning the cichlid with the green net, with the other, he removes the black-light lamp, the cover to the tank. The fish is struggling. I can see his gills puffing out and in, out and in, suffocating. Bruin is suffocating right in front of me. His breathing is rhythmic, but dramatically stifled. The look in his eye is eerily human. I have to peel my eyes away from the tragedy, back up to Mikah's face.

Mikah carefully places the tank's fluorescent light on my desk. The way he neatly rearranges the surrounding items to make room for it starkly contrasts with his actions. It is truly terrifying to watch.

"Please, please, PLEASE! Stop! Mikah! It's suffocating! Put him back!" I scream.

Tears are now running down my face.

Mikah flings the fish out of the net into the paper bag dangling from his arm. He grabs me by the upper arm to force me closer. I refuse to look its direction.

"Look at him! Watch him! Look at him trying to breathe. He's dying," Mikah says calmly, "Look at him!"

He shouts and wraps his hand around the base of my neck, simultaneously forcing my head back around and pushing my face into the bag with the dying fish.

"Get away from me!" Choking back sobs, I cry out, "Get out of my apartment!"

"Okay? Is that what you want? Fine. I'm leaving. You never wanted me here anyway," Mikah says.

Bag in hand, Mikah bounds back into my kitchen. He empties the Cichlid into the sink and turns on the garbage disposal.

"Oh my God, Oh my God. No!" I scream.

I'm walking in circles, trying to clear my mind enough to navigate how to handle the situation. I'm mortified. The crackling of the garbage disposal feels like it's coming from the inside my skull. I look back at Mikah who is now taking dish soap and pouring it into the disposal. Calmly and confidently, he wipes down the inside of the metal sink with the sponge.

I glance over to the fish tank and it's chaos. Water is spilled all down the side of the tank, from the fish's struggling. The water is murky but beginning to settle. The palm tree figurine has been upended and is resting against the front glass. This was Meh, the mini-shark's home, but he is now pushed up against the back of the tank behind a plastic plant. Not one fish is swimming around the tank. The orange and pink female (wife to the blue and yellow male) pokes its head out from its specially bought ceramic house. Three of her babies appear in the makeshift doorway with her.

The tears pour down my face and then suddenly stop. I'm hollow, cold inside. Mikah picks up his leather backpack before he slams the front door so hard the inside of the apartment shakes. I crumple to the floor as Stella sulks out from the closet where she'd been hiding. No kiss attack from Stella today. She lies down next to me on the floor.

DR. BRAUN: JANUARY 5, 2011 (EMAIL)

Mode of Contact: Email
FROM: WHEELER, KALI RAE
SENT: WEDNESDAY, JANUARY 06, 2011 6:06 PM
TO: BRAUN, ALEC J.
SUBJECT: RE: WINTER SUPPORT

I would like to make an appointment as soon as possible.
Sent from my Verizon Wireless BlackBerry

-----Original Message-----
FROM: WHEELER, KALI RAE
SENT: WEDNESDAY, JANUARY 05, 2011 10:31 AM
TO: BRAUN, ALEC J.
SUBJECT: WINTER SUPPORT

Happy New Year Kali
Since I have not heard back from you, I do hope this means you are doing well.
I wanted you to know that I have been able to consult with your other care provider (C.F.), and spoke with her as recently as yesterday. We agreed that it is important for you to resume your work here with me, or someone else if you prefer. We both hope that you will make contact with me in the next two weeks. At the same time, if I do not hear from you in the next two weeks, we also agreed that you should make immediate contact with her since we will both presume that you are no longer interested in seeking services here.
I do hope that you will be able to return to the Center for additional meetings. In case I do not hear from you, here are some community-based referral options...
If you have any questions please do not hesitate to call. And, as always, please recall that we have walk-in appointments between 10am and 4:30pm M-F. We also have a Hotline Service (xxx-xxx-xxxx) available on weekends, holidays and between 5pm and 8am M-F. In case there is an emergency, you can always contact the UCPD, 911, or go to the Hospital ER.
Best wishes,
Alec Braun

DR. BRAUN: JANUARY 6, 2011 (EMAIL)
Mode of Contact: Email
FROM: BRAUN, ALEC J.
TO: WHEELER, KALI RAE
SUBJECT: RE: RE: WINTER SUPPORT

Hi Kali

It is good to hear from you. In order to make an appointment please call the front desk at the telephone number below in order to schedule a meeting within the next two weeks (see previous email on this chain). Thanks.

Best wishes,

Alec J. Braun Ph.D.

DR. BRAUN: JANUARY 13, 2011
MENTAL STATUS
Mood: normal/euthymic and sad/depressed
Affect: congruent with mood and content -Appearance, speech rate and volume, psychomotor activity, orientation, rapport, thought process, perceptions, insight, and judgment are all within normal limits.
HARM TO SELF OR OTHERS
Current Suicidal Concerns?: No, denied current SI.
TREATMENT NOTES
KW arrived in an overtly stable affective state acknowledging frustration about her disappointing audition for spring sing this week. Also addressed dysfunctional and abusive dynamics in her current romantic relationship. Was able to acknowledge co-dependency and need to end the relationship though it would be "hard." Stated that she is still considering the need for counseling regarding her sexual assault experiences. Emotionally processed her unhappy experience at the Newport police station. Support, psychosocial education, and Rx recommendations were provided. KW successfully r/sd [rescheduled] for next week.
GAF: 58
DISPOSITION/TREATMENT PLAN
Focus KW on clear identification of problem areas and beneficial coping strategies. Validate her self-described need for multiple sessions per week and initiate referral to BHS.
FOLLOW-UP APPOINTMENT PLANNED OR SCHEDULED: Yes
INTERVAL UNTIL NEXT APPOINTMENT: Fri 01/21/11

DR. BRAUN: JANUARY 21, 2011 (NO SHOW)
CANCELLATIONS AND NO SHOWS
SCHEDULED DATE OF SESSION: Fri 01/21/11
TYPE: No Show
Signed by Alec Braun Ph.D. on 1/21/2011 10:25:55 AM

DR. BRAUN: JANUARY 21, 2011 (EMAIL)

Mode of Contact: Email
FROM: WHEELER, KALI RAE
SENT: FRIDAY, JANUARY 21, 2011 6:45 PM
TO: BRAUN, ALEC
SUBJECT: RE: TODAY'S 9 AM APPOINTMENT

I was able to make an appointment this morning. I apologize very much for the inconvenience. I have just been sick and slept through my alarm.
I apologize again.
Thank you.
Sent from my Verizon Wireless BlackBerry
-----Original Message-----
FROM: BRAUN, ALEC
SENT: FRI, 21 JAN 2011 09:38:24 -0800
TO: WHEELER, KALI RAE
SUBJECT: TODAY'S 9 AM APPOINTMENT

Hello Kali,

I am writing you regarding our 9am appointment today. I called your mobile phone at approximately 9:15am this morning and left a voicemail. I have not heard back from you. I hope you are doing well.

As you may recall from a previous email, I consulted with your other care provider (C.F.), earlier this month. We agreed that it is important for you to resume consistent work here with me, or someone else if you prefer. We both hoped that you would make contact with me and schedule regular appointments. At the moment, I can hold one appointment time for you on Tuesday (1/25) at 9am. If you cannot make that time please call today and let me know when you are available to speak by telephone in order to discuss your sessions here. If I do not hear from you, please make immediate contact with your other provider as we will both presume that you are no longer interested in seeking services here.

I do hope that you will be able to return to the Center for regular meetings. In case I do not hear from you here again are some community-based referral options:

Best wishes,
Alec

Beneath a Steamer: January 23, 2011

I.
Alive—More than ever,
Yet I'm sinking like a feather.
Or would that float?
Yes, that would float,

II.
Little—Left in the litter.
Feeling—More than a reason,
To light
this lifeless page on fire.

III.
Sleeping.
Careful,
not dreaming.
Writing—
Wait, a
He's reading.
Flying—
Yes!
I'm leading.
Stay!
No!
I'm leaving.
Ssh! The neighbor's hearing!

IV.
Stepping not too close,
But leaning way too far
beyond the rails of the ship, wondering,
What's so bad about churning
beneath a steamer?
If I jumped,
I know you would see me clearer.
They need some more.

V.
Well, I'm bleeding
While he's teething.

And I've been seething
Where's the meaning?
When I'm losing,
And he's winning,
And I'm grinning,
But I'm downing every alcohol in season.
Frowning,
There's not enough space to settle my fear and loathing.

Remember child,
Just stop forgetting.
Just stop believing.

DR. BRAUN: FEBRUARY 9, 2011

MENTAL STATUS
MOOD: normal/euthymic and anxious
AFFECT: congruent with mood and content
Appearance, speech rate and volume, psychomotor activity, orientation, rapport, thought process. perceptions, insight, and judgement are all within normal limits.

HARM TO SELF OR OTHERS
Current suicidal concerns?: No

TREATMENT NOTES
KW arrived in an agitated state. Became disorganized around academic responsibilities in part due to continued relationship with emotionally abusive and controlling bf (e.g., instructing her to not to take her medications, use of profanity and put downs). Acknowledged that she is prone to desire that someone tell her what to do despite abusive guidance by her bf. Has not been adhering to medication protocols due to bfs [boyfriend's] aggressive stance against her taking meds. We discussed need for multiple supports. KW reviewed RTC [rape treatment center] documents and expressed interest in scheduling an appointment. Is also open to consolidating therapy and psychiatry services at BHS [Behavioral Health Services]. KW stabilized by session's end. Agreed to focus on engaging in practices and statements that prioritize her safety.
GAF: 55

DISPOSITION/TREATMENT PLAN
Case plan:
--endorsed decision to be referred to BHS therapy and psychiatry
--accepted Santa Monica RTC hard copy referral information; endorsed willingness to call and schedule an appointment --endorsed willingness to contact current psychiatrist and r/s
--will provide psychoeducation and support regarding boundary/safety management and clinical recommendations
FOLLOW-UP APPOINTMENT PLANNED OR SCHEDULED: Yes

DR. FIASCHETTI M.D. (PSYCHIATRIST): FEBRUARY 16, 2011
Vyvanse 40mg. (See Appendix K.)
Depakote ER 250mg (See Appendix Q.)

DR. BRAUN: FEBRUARY 25, 2011

MENTAL STATUS
MOOD: normal/euthymic, sad/depressed, and anxious
AFFECT: congruent with mood and content -Appearance, speech rate and volume, psychomotor activity, orientation, rapport, thought process, perceptions, insight, and judgement are all within normal limits.

AREAS NOT WITHIN NORMA1 LIMITS
Thought Process & Content: disorganized

TREATMENT NOTES
KW arrived in a stable but distressed state regarding fear of her bf's [boyfriend's] emotional manipulation. Talked at length about the lack of trust, dishonesty, loss of money, and possessiveness in this relationship. Also addressed the derogatory statements that characterize her bf's interactions with her. KW understood how she is being victimized and how alternative choices can enhance her safety. Also understood that the relationship's interfering with academics and her need to begin focusing on prior sexual assaults at the RTC. Discussed boundary setting bxs. Will spend the weekend with her parents and contact the undersigned Monday.
GAF : 55

DISPOSITION/TREATMENT PLAN
Focus on stabilization, interpersonal safety, and firm boundary setting with current bf. KW agreed to spend the weekend with her family for support purposes.

9-1-1; Things Escalate Quickly

It is finals time, and I can't continue to handle situations with Mikah without greatly threatening my academic career and as a result, damaging the rest of my life.

I cannot fail these finals.

Prior to tonight, I've broken up with Mikah twice. It didn't stick. But as the pressure builds around my not nearly finished written finals, and Mikah's obnoxious requests and threats mount, I take immediate action without through of the consequences.

I reiterate the break-up with Mikah again, this time, over the phone. I have several finals due tomorrow and I need to get back to explicating French cinema and John Keats' poetry.

I hang up and transfer all of the energy into my written exams. I am finally able to take a breath without being deflated before I fill my lungs. I get back to my essays, calling Stella over to sit with me while I finish.

Before I can get settled in, I begin receiving text messages.

Within an hour of my breaking it off with Mikah, his text messages take a dark turn. He tells me how is going to kill himself. I block his phone number, but not before responding via text:

Me: Mikah, if you are serious, I think you need to get some help

Mikah is alone at his apartment in West Hollywood sending me very pointed, awful messages. I text Becca, but nothing. The messages continue to come via Facebook, and they are so frightening that in desperation, I find his cousin's phone number and text her to ask if she can call him or get her parents to help in some way.

I have no idea what to do. I don't know anyone else who is close to him who can help. Fearing Mikah is alone and not only contemplating suicide but planning it, I call the police. Another notification pops up on my phone. It's from Mikah, another Facebook message, this one is extremely graphic.

Sobbing on the phone to the 911 operator, I explain the situation. I beg her to check on him somehow. And after a grueling thirty minutes, I get a call back from the police.

"We are outside the address you provided. Which unit number is he staying in?" the officer asks.

"Seven one one. Please don't get him in trouble. I just need to know he's okay," I say.

"Ma'am, we will do whatever we find necessary. Our protocol has nothing to do with you. We need you to stay calm," he says.

"Please, please, please I didn't mean to start a war," I beg. I hear voices yelling in the background.

"I'm going to keep you on the line here. I think this may be him," the officer says. "Sir, we need you to calm down. You are not in trouble," the officer says. Pause "Sir, once again, please let us ask you a couple of questions. Unlock the gate, and we can get this sorted out." The officer comes back on the phone and says to me, "We are going to transfer you back to the operator. We need to ask you some questions too, due to the state he is in. Stay on the line please."

"Please don't get him in trouble. He didn't do anything wrong!" I say. I'm terrified that these cops are not on our team. And the loneliness is overwhelming. The line goes quiet as the officer transfers me to someone else. The silence hurts. A rush of terror washes over me.

Who can I call? Who is there to help me now?

"Hello, ma'am?" a woman's voice asks.

"Yes," I answer.

"I'm from the Los Angeles Police Department; I need to ask you a few questions regarding the person whom you were in a relationship with. He seems to have a couple of things in our system. His response to the wellness check has become irrational," she says.

"No! Please don't do this. He's fine. I just didn't know how to check on him," I say.

The phone notifications cease for a couple of minutes. Thank God. But notifications are now popping up on my Facebook messenger, worse than before. At the same time, his roommate Becca texts me:

Becca: *Go fuck yourself.*

Needless to say, the texts aren't good. They are the most frightening texts I've ever received. She threatens to find and kill me. And then another, from Mikah:

Mikah: *If you ever talk to me again, I'll fucking kill you Dude, I'll fucking kill you.*

Great. So this escalated quickly.

Lost in the messages, I've tuned the operator out, but I now begin to hear her again.

The operator asks me to read her the messages. I read her this one before I realize what it is saying.

"Has he ever been abusive toward you, physically or verbally? Does he own any weapons? Does his family own any weapons? Does your door have a lock that secures? I need you to check that it safely closes while I'm on the phone with you. Did he ever force you to do any drugs? Are you afraid of him?" the 911 operator asks.

The questions are endless, and my defensive answers are probably fueling the fire.

"We are going to have to send a couple of officers to your neighborhood until this calms down. Call this number if you see him anywhere: your apartment, campus, class, anywhere, call us immediately. It's a good idea to stay with friends tonight if you can. We are going to send out a locksmith to change your locks in the morning," she says.

"Okay. Why—" I ask.

"This has nothing to do with you. Ma'am, this man has a record," she says.

"Of what?" I ask.

"I can't disclose that at this time, Ma'am" she says.

"What?" I ask again, as I am flooded with questions all at once, recounting every instance I questioned Mikah's behavior.

"Are you a student at the University?" she asks.

"Yes," I respond, my mind is lost in another world. "Please don' arrest him," I stutter

"Are you currently seeing any kind of psychologist? You can tell us your therapist's name or we can connect you with someone," she continues.

"What?" I ask, nearly panting.

"Do you see a mental health professional at the university?" the operator clarifies.

"Yes. Dr. Braun at the counseling center," I say unthinking.

"Please stay on the line, Ma'am," she says.

How is this real?

I can't breathe.

Only about a minute later, she is back on the line.

"We've connected with your therapist, Dr. Braun, who will have instructions for you regarding your safety getting to and from classes tomorrow," she says.

I begin to cry into the receiver.

"I have finals due tomorrow. This can't happen right now," I say.

I lose the control I've had throughout the call and night.

"Ma'am, you can't take your finals if something happens to you. You need to listen to my instructions and follow them carefully. It would be bad for both of you if something happened. If you need to go outside, I'm going to ask that you disguise yourself," the woman says.

"What, why?!" I ask.

"It's protocol in this type of situation. Ma'am, this man has a record that tells us your safety is in jeopardy right now. Do you understand the instructions for you?" she says.

"Yes," I say.

"Do you have any questions?" the operator asks.

"No...wait, he's not in trouble right?" I ask.

"Unless he does something illegal, he is not in trouble. However, he is not the person you need to be worrying about right now. I need you to protect yourself. We will send officers over shortly to survey the area. I will call you back within the next couple of hours to check in," she says.

What have they found?

Jeremih, Mikah's now former friend, finds me crying on the steps of my apartment the next morning, wearing my dad's old baseball cap and embarrassingly-large sunglasses from high school. I look like the lyrics to a cheesy, "she's a mess," cliché, rock song by Train or somebody. Exhausted from sleep-deprivation and phone calls to the police, counselors, and family members checking on my well-being, Jeremih carries my ninety-pound body up to his apartment at the very top of the driveway. His place overlooks on the sidewalk.

I always love being at Jeremih's place. Especially the giant iguana that is always spectacularly cared for, he is my favorite. It shows me how much of a softy Jeremih is, and it has given me an alibi to hang out over there in days prior. Now it is literally my safe house while the Mikah stuff blows over.

DR. BRAUN: MARCH 2, 2011 (TELEPHONE)
Mode of Contact: Telephone
Returned two calls to Kali today.
A VM requesting a call back was left after the second scheduled t/c [telephone call] attempt. The first call addressed KW's distress regarding her decision to break-up with her bf. Stated that he was initially suicidal. She called the police and they made a wellness check. Had to break down the door. KW learned that he has warrants out for his arrest. Has become fearful. Discovered that he has passwords to her accounts (e.g., Facebook). Encouraged KW to change her passwords quickly. she changed her Facebook account while on the line with the undersigned. Went on to discuss safety options. KW will stay with a neighbor she deems safe. Is also receiving support from her family and her father who is a lawyer. Discussed the benefits of a restraining order. KW's father may be assisting with the latter. Also encouraged KW to contact the RTC. She is not ready at this time. In closing, we discussed how KW might cope with academic responsibilities. KW understands that a letter can be written by the undersigned in order to support her if needed. Also discussed the importance of using 911 from her home phone if needed.
We rs/d [rescheduled] to speak at 5pm today. KW did not respond to this writer's call. VM was left with alternate times to contact this writer tomorrow.

DR. BRAUN: MARCH 3, 2011 (TELEPHONE)
Mode of Contact: Telephone

RTC [rape treatment center] to KW who called while this writer was unavailable. VM was left with options to call back today or at designated times tomorrow.

DR. BRAUN: MARCH 4, 2011 (TELEPHONE)
Mode of Contact: Telephone

KW contacted this writer at approximately 8:30am.
KW stated she feels safe in her apartment and has not decided to initiate a restraining order b/c, "It is too much stress on me. I just want to leave it there and get my homework done." KW stated that her ex-bf is now contacting her and her parents and is being "nice." KW stated that she does not plan to respond to his texts, emails, or vm messages. This writer advised KW that if his bx [behavior] changes and she feels unsafe she can contact 911 and can also call the Hotline. We then confirmed KW's appointment for 3/15 since she is unable to come in on 3/8 at 9am. KW was encouraged to contact this writer if concerns arise before our next meeting.

DR. BRAUN: MARCH 8, 2011 (TELEPHONE/EMAIL)

Mode of Contact: Telephone

VM left on Kali's cell phone service offering appointment times this week. Call back or email response requested.

Mode of Contact: Email
FROM: BRAUN, ALEC J.
TO: WHEELER, KALI RAE
SUBJECT: RE RE: I RECEIVED YOUR TELEPHONE MESSAGE

Hi Kali,

I hope you are doing well.

In light of all the stress you are coping with at this time, please consider coming in this week. I have some times I can offer you on Thursday (3/10) at 9am, 11 am, 1 p.m. or 4 p.m. Please let me know if you are available. Thanks.

Best wishes,
Alec

DR. BRAUN: MARCH 9, 2011 (TELEPHONE)
Mode of Contact: Telephone
VM left at 8:50a.m. requesting call back to r/s this week.

DR. BRAUN: MARCH 9, 2011
Referral to Behavioral Health Institute [BHI]

DR. BRAUN: MARCH 10, 2011

MENTAL STATUS
MOOD: normal/euthymic, hopeless, and angry
AFFECT: congruent with mood and content. -Appearance, speech rate and volume. psychomotor activity, orientation. rapport, thought process. perceptions. insight, and judgment are all within normal limits.

TREATMENT NOTES
KW arrived in an overtly stable affective state but remarking that she has been unable to sleep, feels physically awkward, unable to concentrate and feeling despondent about her life. PHQ-9 elevated at 20. Denied manic sx [symptoms] problems at this time. Also denied SI and SIBs. Still however interacting with ex-bf (e.g. took fish out of the tank and forced her to watch it die). States that she will maintain boundaries when he becomes verbally abusive. The undersigned continues to recommend non-contact, but KW declines. Went on to discuss academic concerns. KW will re-fill the ROIs [release of information]. This writer assisted her with identifying addresses of relevant faculty. KW agreed to pick up letters tomorrow and will contact this writer if she experiences an emotional downturn prior to our next session. At session's end. KW endorsed a BHI referral.

DISPOSITION/TREATMENT PLAN
Continue to contain and stabilize in preparation for BHI referral.

DR. BRAUN: MARCH 14, 2011 (TELEPHONE)

Mode of Contact: Telephone

Received a call from Pam Hendricks requesting an outreach call to Kali. Stated that Kali was crying after being told that she would have to file a request to drop a class since she missed the deadline date for drops. Ms. Hendricks did not observe any indication that Kali was a danger to herself or others.

CONTACT INFORMATION

Spoke with PA who stated that she felt "drained" after making efforts to seek accommodations for her classes. Otherwise, KW gave no indication of risk to herself. Reminded KW that she would be eligible for a letter supporting a drop request. KW then became involved in an off-phone conversation and stated she would call back. Note that PA is scheduled to meet with the undersigned tomorrow.

DR. BRAUN: MARCH 15, 2011 (NO SHOW)
CANCELLATIONS AND NO SHOWS
SCHEDULED DATE OF SESSION: Tues 03/15/11
TYPE: Same Day Cancellation- Rescheduled

DR. BRAUN: MARCH 16, 2011 (EMAIL)
Mode of Contact: Email
FROM: BRAUN, ALEC J.
TO: WHEELER, KALI RAE

Hi Kali,

I hope your week is going well since we last talked.

Since we are running out of sessions for our work together, I left you a voicemail message yesterday about rescheduling with me to address academic concerns you have right now, and to prepare your transition to the new program. The good news is that this program has no session limits and is thankfully located on campus. We will need to move quickly since this program is known for its long waiting list, and I made a special request to get you in.

1. So please call Behavioral Health Institute at 310 ———— and state that you were referred by Dr. Braun to meet with —. They will also need your name, SID, and contact information.

2. Please let me know if you are available to meet next week. I will not be able to meet on Monday but have some morning times on Tuesday, Wednesday, and Friday. I also have some afternoon times on Wednesday and Thursday. Friday is a university holiday.

I look forward to hearing from you, and answering any questions you may have.

Dr. Braun

DR. BRAUN: MARCH 17, 2011 (NO SHOW)
CANCELLATIONS AND NO SHOWS
SCHEDULED DATE OF SESSION: Thurs 03/17/11
TYPE: Cancelled Same Day-Not Rescheduled.††

---

†† I schedule an appointment the evening I recieve his email, but fail to show up for it the next day.

DR. BRAUN: MARCH 18, 2011 (TELEPHONE)
Mode of Contact: Telephone
VM left requesting call back regarding r/sing at CCS [Campus Counseling Center) and BHI

DR. BRAUN: MARCH 23, 2011 (TELEPHONE)
Mode of Contact: Telephone
VM requesting call back from KR r/g previous email and VM.

Meeting the Neighbors

Among the other people I met following the disaster that was Mikah, is Ashlyn, my neighbor, an aspiring vet from the Pacific Palisades, and another neighbor, Felix, a sailor/physicist/drug-enthusiast from Berkeley. His ex-girlfriend is Christina.

The frat-house Sig Ep is next door to my apartment on Carmelina. My kitchen window, the one I jump out to do laundry more easily, is directly below the frat's shower window. It gives the frat-house a bird's eye view of my kitchen. And there is only a two-foot, crumbling brick wall separating their side entrance from our laundry room. We share a Dumpster.

Our building is connected to the frat-house, a good thing, in retrospect, because it keeps me out of the sorority scene. A lot of things did that, but this solidifies that it is not a good idea.

I became friends with the academic guys over there after Ashlyn explained that she used to be a part of that scene and that her best friend lived there. She eventually moved into a frat-house.

I guess that's something you can do?

I have always been good at making friends. I love meeting new people, especially in an environment where we are all playing house on our parents' dime. I feel assured I am doing something correctly by staying up for a week preparing the perfect essay to send to my perverted professors.

Sorry for the perverted part, that is a personal thing. My astronomy professor told me I'd get extra credit if I dressed up as something astronomical for Halloween and sent him the pictures.

Years later, while stumbling through old photographs, I came across a photo of myself and realized that this professor had played me. I was in a yellow sundress with a paper Earth attached to a headband, a star sticker on the outside of my left eye, mouth open, finger pointing up at the Earth on my head. But I did get the extra credit. So there's that.

I remembered taking those pictures because it was right after the incident with Jason. Instead of going back to my apartment after class that day, I drove straight home to Newport with a duffle bag from the night before and a brain that looked like someone lit it up with kerosene and set it on fire. I was out of my mind.

Wandering Into a Frat House

After Mikah and the craziness that ensued, I am forced to stay pretty close to home. The day of the incident, due to Mikah's threatening phone calls, texts and emails, under the guidance of my counselor, (lol wordplay), I have to miss my classes and miss turning in my written finals, the ones I worked on all night into the morning after the ordeal with the police. I got no sleep at all that night.

The days that follow are all fun and games, meeting new people, staying at Jeremih's and talking with friendly strangers, until I get drunk one night and wander next door alone.

I walk through the front door wearing my favorite Rock and Republic jeans Jeans and a cool lacy shawl over my fuchsia bikini top.

"Hey girl!" Kevin calls out. He stretches the "r" like a "grrrrrrrr." He's holding a red cup but isn't overwhelmingly drunk. "Kali! Come cut our hair again!"

He is referring to the time they believed in my ability with a buzzer and allowed me to turn a good twelve members of their fraternity into mini-Jaxx Moreaus. Remembering it makes me laugh.

"Come! We have Jungle Juice for you!" Kevin says.

We pass the first bedroom, and I run into Braiden, an innocent-looking member of the squad, whom I always took kindly to because he had a kind face.

He was like a purebred golden retriever puppy. I had never dated anyone my age, especially not like him. But he is cute.

Ashlyn laughed when I revealed my crush to her.

"He's super nice, but a total nerd," she said.

I black out almost immediately and wake up in bed next to Gavin. He has on my favorite pair of Rock and Republic jeans.

"We switched!" Gavin says, pointing to Braiden, who is wearing my fuchsia bikini tied around his head. They are laughing. I look down quickly and am relieved to be wearing someone's baggy t-shirt.

"I want to go home. Please take my jeans off," I say.

I look around at the disgusting room: bottles everywhere, stained carpet. Through a door, I can see the shower, the one that looks right down into my apartment window.

"We watch you from there," Says one of the guys on the bed.

"That's disgusting."

I feel a chill jump down my spine and realize it's not just because I'm terrified about the situation.

"Why am I wet?"

The boys laugh. There are far more people in this bedroom than I realized.

"You were dirty. So we made you take a shower." Kevin says.

The two laugh together. The frat brothers won't answer my questions.

"Give me my jeans, Gavin. I want to go home."

"No. Make me."

I feel like I'm in prison. I've lost the ability to perceive the bigger picture. I feel like I am being forced to stay in this disgusting prison of a bedroom.

There are guys everywhere, standing in front of the door, lying on the bunkbeds… I am disoriented, not sure how much time has passed since I arrived… And then it hits me, I can make a run for it! Except I've lost my keys, shoes, purse, wallet and I've yet to find my phone. My jeans and bikini are being held from me as collateral.

I can climb through the window.

I push past the laughing Gavin.

"Kali, you're not done here!"

The Fraternal Instincts: Spring 2011

Take her to a higher place where the flowers die
and the arrows flow
Cupid's bow broke in two disbelief.
It's unbelievable, the Phoenix arose from the ashtray.
When you're sucking for bucks You're in a rush
Money is calling, Go!
Then you're left among the dust and the others in the room-- the cold floor,
your Indian style position,
the empty beers scattered amongst glass shards.
A tired smile makes an appearance then dissipates and a neon sign across the way says something like...
something like...
Basically, it says I represent brotherhood and getting laid, premarital sex and candy.
Then there are the nightstands.
Many nightstands, to be exact,
for the many nights of the year filled with women, only can use 'em once.
The forgotten names,
forgotten articles of several scents,
they are in a drawer not allowed to reunite with their sorority sisters.
Not allowing notches 1, 2, 3, 69 to retrieve
What's left of me.
You're thinking provocative.
I'm thinking overseas
reactors are exploding in Japan
Yet saki and sushi remain goddamn free!
The man cannot afford these generosities but provides them to her willingly.
Ah my little Geisha. Drink up sweetie.
Whetting her palate for tonight's debauchery.
He's yearning for another notch to intensify the meaning behind this worldwide fraternity.
Suck for bucks?
I suck on rubber ducks, alongside bubbles
soon to be wrapped like candies
around privates much too much for the straight-edged camera flashing in front.
Even at three,

in the bathtub with Barbie and chew toys,
so intensely suck-ably free.
Why do we all want to suck on things?
After I get my shot, Mommy, Dr. Barnett will give me a sucker.
Awkward?
Dwell on this for a moment or two,
Intensify that smell your senses cannot define. Get on the bus lonely Figga!
It's an F not an N
viii
Fox not Never
Never rearrange Figga
For it can be repeated in rap songs
If you're one of them.
But how come you can say it like you're the rapper's best friend Why can't I say it then?
English
ENlish
Elish.
I-T apostrophe S
Not a bad dream lovely,
It's a realization
DreAM or PM
I'm really not too sure.
If you're looking for poetry I've got the treasure,
Fall asleep in a field of poppy weeds or seeds because they'll grow.
Opium will take you there…
You can sit next to the sign and feel just like the other lonely people gazing through window pains of use and neglect-ion.

Through the Window

It's dark outside, black-dark. I have no idea what time it is, but it's late. It isn't morning yet, though. There isn't that overwhelming feeling that you've overstayed your welcome, disrespected the natural rhythm of time, but bypassing the time you were supposed to be sleeping.

I'm stumbling back from the fraternity house. I make it to the plants in front of my apartment, shifting backward a bit to find my stability. My body's wavering momentum is staggering. Everything is spinning.

I'm trying to find the flow of things, but it's like being on the subway. You feel stable and then:

BOOM!

You realize why you are holding so tightly to the pole in the center, and you nearly fall face first into the person in front of you.

My keys are God knows where, and my dignity, well, that left a long time ago. It looks like it's time to break into my apartment via the front window.

"Kali! Kali!" her voices wobbles, "Say something! I saw you fall off the ledge! Are you okay?" Ashlyn's voice breaks. "I'm calling nine one one. Please don't be mad at me." I hear her voice in the distance. "Hello? Yes. Hi. I have an emergency. My friend Kali just fell and hit her head... No.

No." I let her voice fade into the darkness. My eyelids won't open when I try, so I let it go. My head is throbbing.

Am I on the ground? Where am I? Was I hit by a car? Crap...the driveway of my apartment. The window...

"Don't call the cops," I mumble and give up.

I'm so tired.

The words I'm thinking don't seem to come out right; I can't form sentences.

"Her eyes are rolling back in her head. They're closed...mostly. Please get here quickly. Okay..." Ashlyn says.

Silence.

Kali! Kali! Stay here! Open your eyes!" Ashlyn shouts. She is shaking me, and now her voice is panicked.

Relax, Ashlyn. It's all just fine. You don't need to worry all the time, we are okay, always.

"Yes! No! No! Yes! I saw it! Okay...okay," Ashlyn says into the phone. "The ambulance is on the way, Kali," she says to me. Her voice is closer than before; she must be kneeling next to me.

"Why do you have to be so crazy, girl?! You could have slept at my place! Where were you tonight anyway!?... If you were next door, I am going to be so mad at those guys. It's not even funny."

The familiar silence envelops me.

"Wake up! I have mac and cheese!" Ashlyn says.

I love mac and cheese.

"I am, I am trying. She's not responding to me." Ashlyn maintains her composure despite being audibly terrified. "No Ash—" I mumble.

Sirens echo in the driveway of the apartment building. The ambulance arrives, and I'm too drained to be embarrassed. The bright lights behind my lids remind me of how exposed I am, lying out there like a DaVinci painting.

I can't feel my body. After tonight, I don't want to anyway.

The memory of waking up at Sig Ep sends pangs down my back, much worse than any pain from a fall.

All twenty apartments in the building surround and overlook this U-shaped driveway.

They are all watching, and I have an oversized men's t-shirt on, no pants.

I give up trying to bargain with my mind, to mentally battle the feeling.

"Kali? We hear you took quite the fall tonight. Is that correct? I need you to speak to me, hon… You've got to open up your eyes for me," a woman says. I blink. A female paramedic kneels into view and says, "Can you tell me your name?"

I shift my blank stare to meet hers.

"Kali. I'm Kali," I say.

Several things happen at once. One man is at my feet, straightening my legs out by the ankles and latching them to something sturdy. Someone is cradling my neck.

Another paramedic is taking my vitals and the woman speaking is holding my hand in hers like a paw.

I try to move my head, but it's already fastened to something.

When did that happen?

"Are you taking any medications, Kali?" she asks.

"Synthroid—" I say.

Things fade out again.

"What was that, Kali? Kali. Kali, we need you awake," the paramedic says.

"I can help with that," Ashlyn volunteers, "There's a few. She's on Lyrica…"

Not anymore, Ashlyn…

Her voice fades as a new paramedic approaches. I become very aware that I am not wearing pants as the men strap me to the backboard. Their hands are all over me, and I can't do a thing.

Not for the first time tonight, my legs bristle with goose bumps in fear.

I can feel the straps around my naked thighs, and I want to scream. Lying there, completely immobile but acutely aware that men are standing above me, staring down at me. One guy is calling my parents, but the other two are talking so casually it tips me over the edge.

The woman paramedic is talking to Ashlyn separately. Their voices are distant now.

Where did these guys take me?

My eyes open quickly: a subconscious safety valve.

He looks familiar. I know that face… Wait, he looks just like… No! I know this guy! Wait! Stop! I know this paramedic!

"No! No! No! Get away from me!" I scream.

I'm struggling to release myself from the straps on the backboard. The paramedics who walked back to their truck come running. I can hear their boots reverberate off the walls of the building as they strike the pavement.

"Get him away from me! Are you Beau? Are you Beau? Are you Beau!" I shout.

In my frenetic, utterly hopeless panic attack, I've managed to scrape my shoulder badly on the asphalt driveway, unable to get out of the restraints.

The paramedics surround me once more to hold the board flat back onto the pavement.

I'm in a sort of hellish reality. He is everywhere.

"Get him away from me!" I shout.

"It's me, Beau," the new paramedic says.

"Get him away from me!" I scream, in utter terror. It's the definition of blood-curdling.

How could he be here! How could he have followed me here? No! No! No! Get him away, someone please protect me. He's going to do it. He's going to do it again!

I'm shaking now.

"Don't touch me! Please don't let him touch me. Get your hands off of me. Please, someone, help me stop him," I plead with the three paramedics who strapped me down.

"Sandra!" the guy holding my neck shouts.

"Please don't let him touch me. Please!" I shout. I look for assurance in this paramedic's eyes. I lock gazes with him.

Please protect me. Please stand up for me.

"Wait in the truck," the paramedic holding my neck shouts to Beau.

"Who is Beau?" Beau says as he retreats.

Sandra is back in my frame of vision. She says, "I was talking with your friend Ashlyn. She may have saved your life you know... Now we need you to calm down, so we can get you into the ambulance and to the hospital. I will ride with you. But it's very important that you calm down."

A moment later Beau and Paramedic 3 approach me.

"His name is Sam. Here's his license." The pseudo-Beau apologizes. But the damage is done.

"Get him away from me," I repeat. My chest fills with anger as the tears dry, sticky on my cheeks. Beau recedes.

Paramedic 2 keeps his gaze locked with mine and says, "We are going to get you into the ambulance and take you to the hospital now."

They recite in unison: "One. Two. Three...Up..."

Before I can process things, I'm lifted up and I hear a click. The table shifts into motion. The gravel underneath the wheels jumbles the ride.

I can't feel any part of my body except for the soft sheet on my thighs. I wiggle my fingers. They are cold. I hope I didn't paralyze myself.

The siren is muted, but audible inside the ambulance as we speed down the street to the hospital. I watch Sandra bounce up and down with the pitted streets of Westwood.

What happened tonight? Where are my jeans? Where is my bathing suit top?

I walked over to the frat house to tan and study with my so-called friend around midday. Now I am in this an ambulance in a boy's t-shirt.

What happened? I had a plan.

The fluorescent lights of the emergency room hurt as I strain my eyes to find my parents standing to the left of my bed. The man with the clipboard walks in.

"Good news. It doesn't look like you have a concussion. How many fingers am I holding up?" the doctor asks.

"Four. Two. Umm three?" I say.

"Nice! The last one was a trick." The doctor laughs looking for a reaction, but my face is fixed.

"Why are my parents here?" I ask.

"Oh God, Kali," my mother says. She turns toward the door, obnoxiously throwing her arms to her sides.

"Michelle, come on," my dad says.

"Because you got fucking drunk. And ya fell down a flight of stairs onto your head. That's why we're here. Because we're your parents," my mom says.

"Cool," I say.

"Your friend Ashlyn saw you from her balcony," a female nurse says, "She watched you fall off your steps and smack your head on the concrete. She called us, and when we took your vitals, it was decided you needed to be taken here for evaluation."

"Can I go home?" I ask.

"Yes, as soon as the IV is finished," the nurse says.

"Saline?" I ask.

"Yes, saline. I will sign your release form as soon as it's finished," she says.

I know my dad won't be happy with that decision. The saline will take the edge off of the hangover I am meant to feel in the morning.

"Okay, get dressed then," my mom is pissed. "Where are your clothes? Do you even have clothes, Kali?"

"Please leave me alone," I say.

"I'm leaving, Atticus. You can deal with this," my mom says to my dad before grabbing her purse and walking out. My father follows after lingering a moment.

I don't have any clothes, and I don't have any idea why.

Ashlyn walks in. "You okay?"

"Yeah, I'm good. My mom's being a bitch, though," I say.

"She's just worried about you," Ashlyn says.

"Yeah, whatever," I say.

"Well, I'm going to go home. I drove my car behind you guys. I'll call you in the morning. Love you, girl!" Ashlyn says.

"Thanks, Ashlyn," I say.

Looking up at the saline bag, I wonder if anything happened the night before. Other than falling down the stairs and hitting my head on the concrete, did anything happen at the frat-house? I quickly try and retrace my night, but can only get as far as being asked if I will trade jeans with Gavin. I agreed, but he didn't fit into my Rock and Republic jeans. They were my favorite ones. I winced as I drunkenly watched the stitched crowns on the back pockets stretch, as he danced around with a handle of Jack Daniels.

That is the only part I remember. It is all black after that: a void of just…nothing. There were a lot of people wherever we were, but I don't remember where this room was located.

The nurse walks in to take down the saline IV. She carefully removes the IV and replaces it with a cotton ball and bandage.

"Thanks. Can I wear the gown home…and the socks?" I ask.

The nurse smiles warmly. "They're yours… Where are your clothes?"

"I don't know. I had this guy's shirt on, but they cut it off," I say.

"You were barefoot too? I don't see a belongings bag for you," the nurse says.

"Yeah. After…" I begin.

She looks up quickly. "You want to talk?"

"No. My dad is here. Please just let me go home. I don't remember anything," I say.

"Okay," she says and moves away from the bed so that I can stand. "Just know that if you do start to remember anything, anything, you should come back here. Or just go to your doctor. But tell someone. Do you have a therapist?"

"Yeah," I respond.

"Tell him. I overheard you had been at a frat-house right before the fall?" she says.

"Yeah, it's next door to me," I reply.

She frowns. "You really ought to talk to someone, but I understand." She hands me her card. "If you need anything, call me, I mean it."

I'm too upset, humiliated, to make eye contact. "Thank you," I say.

"Be safe, you are too young," the nurse says.

"We're here," my mom says, irritated, when we arrive at my apartment.
"Thanks," I say.
"Do you need help walking?" my dad asks.
"No. I'm fine," I say.
"Please call us in the morning," he says. His eyes are unusually glassy.
"Yeah, okay. Will do," I say. I slam the door to my dad's truck.

I must have been in the ER for a while before they arrived since they drove all the way up from Orange County after the paramedics called. I grab the bottom of the hospital gown and twirl it to the front, so I don't flash my parents as I walk past the dark windows of the other tenants. The pavement is cold and rough on my bare feet. It's early morning now. The sky looks deep red.

I can feel again. I feel broken, again. I've felt this feeling before. But never in front of witnesses, especially not my parents.

I've never felt worse about myself than I do walking away from my dad's truck in a hospital gown and socks that I had to borrow from the ER's supply. I lied to my parents about having keys.

I watch my dad drive around the driveway and make the turn left down Carmelina. I then climb through the window.

Stella bounds across the apartment. Her enthusiasm shuts me down. I can't hold myself up anymore, and I crumple onto the ground, holding Stella's collar.

I will never speak of what happened tonight…ever.

They weren't supposed to see this.

Stella's collar is soon soaked in tears.

I lay myself down on the floor in a fetal position. Stella gets into her crate and curls up too. I guess I'll sleep on the floor tonight.

A Paramedic's Mistake: Spring 2011

When things begin to make nonsense,
milky marble-eyes roll aimlessly.
The ambulance sounds
finally,
but help has far from arrived.
Jumbled voices,
Synchronized movements,
And men quick to demand Don't talk sweetheart. As she asks, Am I too heavy to lift?
No one is there.
 The backboard would be of no use, As the paramedic's mistake happened to unlace
rotten stitches,
 far too troubling to be dealt with unequipped. So he left her a victim
And not a patient.
 He thought it would comfort her to make it clear
that he was the one to steal her life, her dignity,
 and her self-worth--
tumbling her chastity ring between nasty fingers, wearing it without permission
leaving it mangled,
and now she feels strangled.
 No butterfly Band-aids will suffice for the terror she should not have had to experience from a lousy paramedic with a heart of ice.
 So, now there's gravel digging into a numb face, She's struggling to escape.
Caught off guard as he pulls out his id,
Nothing changes in her vivid memories.
 She's screaming as they strap her down, and jab her with a thorny IV.
They cut her clothes off with ease.
 She's stripped.
 Not Him Not Him Not Him.
 He should've read the look on her face--
the seething for him to tell her another name: one that promised not to do the same, one that promised to keep her safe.
An id,
Next to nothing
He embedded himself within a scarred memory.
And so to her,
her attacker attacked again.

Get Away Get Away
Not Him!

The scar remains smacked upon her chest. A reminder of the night she fell,
more than just down the steps.
A reminder of the night she fell,
    Back into the arms of the aggressor.
    Any given sedative could've eased her pain, But the paramedic wanted to play games under a life-threatening pseudo name.

EMERGENCY ROOM: MARCH 28, 2011
EMERGENCY ROOM VISIT

[Intake Notes]
   TIME: 2:30 a.m.
   HISTORY FROM: friend and EMT
   CHIEF COMPLAINT: witnessed trip and fall over 3 stairs, admits drinking etoh tonight, on full c-spine precaution.
   History: 19 y/o student fall backwards onto concrete from three steps off ground. Hit head "hard" according to witness. Per Ashlyn, pt. had been drinking at fraternity.
   PHYSICAL EXAM: bruises, abrasions, rash [from concrete]
   OTHER: anxious

[Discharge Notes]
   ENCOUNTER SUMMARY
   FAMILY WAITING: YES
   OUTCOME: Discharge
   LOCATION: Home
   CONDITION: Satisfactory
   CHIEF COMPLAINT: Fall Injury - witnessed trip and fall; + etoh
   DIAGNOSIS: Closed Head Injury, Alcohol (ETOH) Intoxication
   CUSTOM NOTES: You were seen for head injury after a fall while intoxicated. Your exam is benign and is safe to be discharged home. Avoid alcohol consumption. Follow up with the student center in one week. Return if you have worsening headache or nausea, vomiting.

DR. BRAUN: MARCH 30, 2011 (EMAIL)
Mode of Contact: Email
FROM: BRAUN, ALEC
TO: WHEELER, KALI

Hi Kali,

I hope the spring break was restful and restorative for you.

I remain hopeful that you will schedule a meeting with me within the next 10 days so that we can discuss your needs and the referral I have arranged for you. As you know, I have attempted to contact you on multiple occasions during and after final exams and have not received an email or call-back from you. I understand that things can get quite busy. At the same time, please recall that I continue to be in contact with your previous provider, and we still have an understanding that if you are unable to meet with me consistently, you will return to your ongoing work with her (see email below). Or if you like, please feel free to contact me regarding the on-campus referral option I discussed with you, or the other referral options in the email below.

I do sincerely look forward to reconnecting with you. If we do not talk by telephone or meet in my office within the next ten days, I will presume that you are no longer interested in our services and will advise your current provider that you will now be working with her. In either case,

Best wishes,

Dr. Braun

Mammoth

I am invited by a fellow English major, Jakob, to come with him and the ski/snowboard team to Mammoth. I think it is a good idea to branch out, make new friends, and Jakob assures me that it is okay to be an intermediate boarder.

Today is a new day! Time to snowboard like a champion!
I get out of bed the morning of the trip, with a renewed excitement for the adventure ahead. I'll be traveling…with a stranger…to the mountains that hold a huge part of my childhood memories. I love it. I thrive in impossibly uncomfortable situations. They are a challenge, a dare.

The ride up is not that eventful. Jakob's friend in the passenger seat pulls out a pipe almost immediately. We haven't even gotten to the freeway yet. We take turns taking hits.
This is a mistake, I realize quite quickly. I start talking, of course, about anything and everything. And then, I start apologizing for talking so much and then for apologizing for talking so much and—(it goes on a bit like that).
"Sorry Kali, I forgot to tell him you don't smoke sativa," Jakob says.

"Oh my God! Is that it? Okay, cool, I feel a bit better knowing that I'm not a crackhead. Again, I'm sorry for talking so much, you guys—" I say.

Soon enough, I'm asleep.

It is not long before we are pulling into a snow-filled parking lot at the local grocery store to buy food. I am overwhelmed with trying to figure out what I need to buy. I take hints from the other two girls who are with us. They are a lot more confident than I am for some reason. I buy a box of oatmeal and some water to fit in.

Jakob said he'd take care of everything and so I allow him to arrange the trip without any info. I am thinking catered, luxurious cabin, to be honest.

I am in for a treat.

Jakob is the only person I know, and he said that people on the board team could bring guests. I agreed to come, expecting not to be his one and only guest on the trip, treated like what feels like a claim-stake.

The three-bedroom mountain home is crawling with college kids.

I look for a place that isn't covered in couples making out, people about to have sex, or someone's Patagonia sleeping bag, perfectly laid-out before anyone has arrived (how did they arrange this?). The only thing I find is a very tiny closet, maybe six by three feet. It has a sliding door that closes. It isn't a full coat closet, but is probably deep enough to hold a vacuum.

I step over the couples who were chatting in their sleeping bags, but are now making out in one sleeping bag and using the other as a comforter.

The bed is reserved for six, not kidding, guys. The floor on the other side of the bed is home to three more sleeping bags, two parallel and one running the other direction to face the door. (Talk about bad feng shui with the sleeping bag placement.)

There are people everywhere; on all of the couches, and both of the beds (there are only two). The den is like one big sorority house, piles of purses and bags and there's one community shower. It is beyond disgusting.

This isn't the cabin I imagined.

I am freaked out, to say the least. So I get drunk, very drunk.

I drink everything in sight: wine, vodka, beer, more boxed wine, more beer. I end up teaching the two girls I came up with to dance. We proceeded to perform said dance, turns, booty pops and all, over and over and over again.

I pass out on the couch occupied by an awkward tall dude who seems infatuated with every word I speak. This works in my favor as he has claimed the couch and I want somewhere to sleep.

We wake up before 6 a.m. the next day, and I am trashed. I can hardly move.

How will I make it through the day? Let alone snowboard.

The first run is when I realize this isn't gonna be fun. I'm dead last and the awkward girls from the night before are even more confident on the slopes than they were in the grocery store. They both glide down the mountain on skies.

The moguls are the end of the trip for me. Three runs in, post-moguls, I throw up in my mouth, trailing behind the team of six, all skiers.

I am weak in the legs. I head inside to sleep, boots already rubbing blisters. It is noon and I am done with this trip. I want to sleep and then I want out.

Now.

If I was done last night, I am completely finished today.

That night, I manage to muster enough courage to face everyone. It is impossible to hide from the forty guests stuffed into the tiny, two-story house anyway. I throw back a couple of shots of liquid courage with a random creep near the Pac-Man machine as I exit the bedroom/broom closet I am sleeping in.

Time to socialize again.

I want to sleep so badly by midnight that I curl up at the foot of the only bed upstairs. There is a hefty man under the covers, completely knocked out. No big.

I think it is safe until he asks me what I am doing and allows me to get under the sheets. It isn't long until he starts rubbing my leg.

Eventually, he gets the picture and leaves me alone to sleep.

The second morning, I am even more so trashed than the first. I cannot walk straight. There is no way I'm getting to my snowboard gear: none.

My world is spinning.

Jakob tells me that I can't stay at the house because everyone is leaving.

To ride back with him, I have to come with them to the mountain for the day. So I sit in the hot, sweaty car the entire day, waiting for them to finish skiing so we can drive home. I spend my day feeling like I am coming off some sort of hard drug. I am so embarrassed when I see the group finally walking toward the car. My head is a mess from stress hormones. It has been one of the worst weekends of my life.

I cannot figure out why my head is so all over the place. It is probably because no normal person would sit in a car next to the slopes for an entire day in order get a ride back to LA from her "friend" who turned out to be more of a horny dick when he realizes he is definitely going to stay in the friend zone, forever.

I cannot wait to get back home, sleep, shower and never do any group trip ever again. Note to self: Add group trips with Jakob to Things NOT to Do list.

DR. BRAUN: APRIL 7, 2011 (NO SHOW/TELEPHONE)
CANCELLATIONS AND NO SHOWS
SCHEDULED DATE OF SESSION: Thurs. 04/07/11
TYPE: NO SHOW.
Mode of Contact: Telephone
VM left regarding call back regarding today's missed appointment. Reiterated that transfer of care would be turned over to her current psychiatrist of I did not hear from her. Best times to contact the undersigned either today or tomorrow were provided.

His Eyes: Lapses Part 1

I feel the car surge and stop. I've been half asleep for most of the drive out of Mammoth.

"Okay, wake up! We're halfway!" Jakob says. He turns around from the driver's seat. "Bathroom time!"

It's almost dusk outside.

I look at the two other back-seaters nestled up together in the middle and far right spaces of Jakob's Volvo. Amanda looks like a child. Her mascara is smeared under her lashes, baby hairs pressed against her forehead.

"I'm good" she says, sleepily and re-acquaints her shoulder with the side of the door.

She looks more comfortable than I've been for the past four years.

Things are hazy around me. I note that it is not a haze coming from the small pipe Nick in the passenger seat is placing in the center cup-holder.

I feel weightless, but heavy, and uncoordinated all at once. Nick energetically pops out of the car and walks toward the gas station. I feel dissed by his distant attitude in such an intimate setting. Sleeping is a vulnerable state.

I push open the door on my side and my pillow and prized Marc Jacobs purse thunk to the cement. My cell phone smacks the ground and tumbles under the car. Jakob crouches under his Volvo to grab my phone.

Damn he is always so nice to me.

"Thanks!" I say.

My eyelids are heavy as I place my things back inside the car. Michael in the middle seat crawls out behind me.

We walk together into the gas station store somewhere in Barstow. There is one unisex bathroom. Nick exits and smirks as he walks past me. I fumble with the mini cereal boxes waiting for the vacant sign.

After tip-toeing around the dirty bathroom and enduring the mini thigh workout it takes to pee in a public bathroom, I push the heavy door open with my elbow. Jakob is next in line so I take a seat at a table near the cement trash-can by the commercial push-bar exit of the gas station. I watch the wind outside whisk dirt into the air.

An evil-looking man approaches the gas station. His eyes are dark, eyebrows furrowed, his criminal body language and angular movement strike me. His bomber jacket and Levi's aren't anything scary, but the white baseball cap is odd. His lips are thin and pursed.

I'm struck by the physical reaction I have as I look down at the goosebumps on my arm.

CLUNK

I look up to meet the gaze of the man. His eyes are triangular and steel gray. I've never seen anything like them. He is angry with me. I see it in his eyes. And then I fall into the terror of his glance. He doesn't rush to look away, but keeps eye contact from the time he notices me until he presses open the door to the gas station. He craned his neck to keep staring before jolting his head forward to smash the door open.

His glance stays in my mind as he turns away.

Maybe I have seen that before.

I sink into this thought. His pair of steel-colored eyes remain fixed in front of mine. They are penetrating and repulsive, demeaning, manipulative and relentless.

I am helpless as I'm thrown back to someplace in my mind. Things are enclosed and the lights are dim in a space where I can't find the exit. His disembodied eyes hover in front of mine, staring, hating me animalistically.

My heartrate skyrockets as I watch the baseball cap bob above the aisle of junk food, passing the last aisle, there he is again. Having already turned his head slightly to the left to stare at me as he exits, he jolts his gaze forward and slams against the push door with both hands. I swallow my breath, heart racing.

Black

"Kali Rae! Can. You. Hear. Me?" Jakob is kneeling in front of me. His hands gripping my shoulders. I move my head slowly to meet his gaze.

"That guy was so scary…his eyes," I say.

"She's awake!" Jakob shouts to Amanda who trudges half-asleep through the gas station doors, looking motherly and worried.

"What the heck, girl!" Amanda says, standing, arms-crossed, leaning into one hip. "I couldn't get you to move. You were staring at me and not responding for like five minutes. Are you okay?"

"Wait…seriously? I was just sitting thinking about his eyes…that guy…" I say.

"That was the weirdest fucking thing," Jakob says. He's looking away from me and down at the ground. I've never seen him so thrown. "Here, let's get out of here. Can you walk?"

"Yeah of course, I was just thinking and that man was so…" I say and stand up. Jakob rushes around to hold my arm.

"I don't know what just happened. But let's go home," Jakob says, basically carrying me to the car.

"Wait, I was looking at you and not responding?" I ask.

"Yeah. But…like…not at me, through me," Jakob walks me forward more quickly. Amanda moves to the other side of me. "It's like you couldn't see or hear me. Your eyes would occasionally move, like you were watching someone. I was shaking you… Honestly scariest shit I've ever seen… I didn't want to leave you, but had to get Amanda to see if she could help. I didn't take my eyes off you as I ran to the car… It was like…"

We're back at the car now as Jakob's story becomes distant and begins to reverberate off something.

"Kali!" he shouts.

"Yes! Here!" I respond quickly.

"Geez, it looked like you were doing it again. Just get in the car. Let's get home," Jakob says.

"What is up with you, man?" Amanda rubs my shoulders like a boxing coach.

"Did you guys see that guy? I just saw his eyes…" I say.

I wake up to Amanda nudging me harshly. "Wake up, Sleepy Head, we don't know your apartment address," she says almost obnoxiously, but that is her default tone. She is president of the club for God's sake.

"Uhh…Carmelina," I say, "I don—" and pass out for a moment again.

I hear Jakob's familiar, worried voice. "Kali! We need you to wake up and tell us where to go."

"Oh sorry. Um…four sixteen or something. Just go to Sig Ep," I answer.

"Dude I'm not taking you to a frat-house right now like this," Jakob says.

"It's next door," I say and half pass out for the next few blocks.

I am so dizzy. I try to put the ex-boyfriend's sweater I have been using as a pillow, back into my neon-orange backpack. I almost fall into the gutter.

"Here ya go!" Jakob's tall friend has removed my luggage from the trunk and placed it on the curb.

"Oh thanks. Thank you," I say.

I bust into my apartment, throw my things on the floor. I go to grab my phone to text my mother that I am indeed, alive.

Shit.

I've lost my phone.

Driving to Get Stella: Lapses Part 2

It is early afternoon when I wake up from the daze of the journey home the prior day. The sun is obnoxious beaming through the window. It is oddly lonely in here. Stella's cage is open, deserted. My clothing is everywhere from my attempt to unpack last night. This was before realizing I left my phone in Jakob's car. Thank God Amanda lives up the street and walked it down to me.

I grab my phone tighter as I see the messages displayed for the first time since yesterday early afternoon:

Mom: Where are you?!
Mom: Are you heading back?
Mom: Please Answer me.
Mom: Are you coming to Newport to pick up Stella?
Isaak: Yo Kali, mom's freaking out, where are you
Isaak: Please call us as soon as you get this, we have no idea if you're okay.
Shit.

I try to answer a few of the important ones.

I hate texting.

I have a panicking mother wondering if I am alive mixed in with messages from drunk friends and a bunch of new friends with numbers I don't recognize asking vague, sometimes rhetorical questions.

The list of messages is so mixed up, it's overwhelming, especially without my morning coffee. I turn the phone off altogether and throw on some Ugg boots. I had fallen asleep in sweats and a hoodie and made no effort to change.

Time to get Stella back from my parents.

I jump on the 405, and its emptiness is glorious.

It's a much-needed relief.

On the way to Newport, there are a few incidences where I have to roll down the windows and blast music to keep myself awake. I didn't take my Synthroid for the length of the trip, and I am in a state beyond tired. I know how I feel, but I am not aware that I can't control it.

I press on, thinking I can sleep for as long as I want once I arrive.

Suddenly, the man with the steel eyes morphs into a clear and terrifying image, and I stop analyzing why I am tired. I shake out of the trance as I drift into the next lane.

I swerve and the car levels out.

Holy. I've got to stop.

I pull over at the next exit and end up in an area I've never seen before.

Is this Anaheim? Gross.

I sleep for twenty minutes and wake up feeling alright. Still a while to go. I set out. The freeway stretches out before me, but my ability to stay awake dwindles. To compensate, I drive faster. I need to get home, immediately, and sleep.

I safely make it to Newport and am greeted by an excited puppy-dog and a worried mother.

"Kali!" my mom shrieks. I hear the clank of Stella's collar.

"Hellllooooooo," I say, sounding just like my grandmother. I'm greeted with a very tight hug.

"Stella's excited to see her mommy! She wouldn't stop whimpering the other day," my mom says.

"How are you, Mom?" I ask. I get up from my crouching position to hug her again.

"I've been worried about you, Angel." She hugs me again, "Two nights in a row I woke up and started throwing up in fear."

A cold chill runs down my spine as she continues.

"Did something happen to you?" she can read my mind, but I won't ever admit that.

"Mom, a lot has happened. But no, nothing out of the ordinary this weekend, just a lot of snowboarding," I lie. "I did forget my Synthroid though. I've never been this tired. I feel like someone is standing above me pressing down on my head, closing my eyelids."

"Want me to make you coffee?" she asks.

"Yes! Thank you. I've got to get back up there for class by eleven," I say.

"Yikes, okay. Have a few cups of coffee first." Staring at me, she adds, "Maybe three. You look really tired. I think you should take the day off. Sleep here and recuperate; it's been a rough week."

I wish, but no way. My professor grades on attendance, and I'm already failing for not doing the "right" kind of assignment for him. He's square, and I'm rectangular. We don't get along, so I need to make it to class, especially after missing the day before Mammoth.

After unloading all of the ski gear I borrowed from the family stock (a.k.a. from the big box labeled "ski stuff" with assorted things from ski pants to beanies, goggles, and disposable toe warmers) my mom helps load Stella into the spacious back seat of my Range Rover.

We take off, and Stella is happy as a clam. It feels good to have her with me again. I smile to myself in gratitude. She has stuck with me through everything. After attempting to get herself into the passenger seat for a good ten minutes, she finally decides to take a nap on the floor behind the driver's seat.

Till Morning's Light: Spring 2011

Wake up
Wake up 6ZFG373
Wake up darling
Wake up

Motor Vehicle Accident,
MVA as the report concluded,
Try and decipher number 373—
Who's still contemplating,
waiting on the figure
dressed in black.
He comes,
he goes,
rest he brings,
the rest…
no living knows.

Wake up
Wake up 6ZFG373
Wake up
It's not your time yet…

Man's best friend is alive and well.
It must be 373's time to go.

Goodnight sunrises that woke me up too late
Goodnight heartache flooded by bad music
Night night nightmares, only breathing now due to my turtle nightlight—
the terrors you bring stick me a hell of in between
But now I am in limbo, Goodbye.

Swept away sturdy,
leaving her doggy behind.

Stella, remember,
you don't ever have to put on the red light.
Wake up…
Wake up…
Wake up…

Thank you lord for another day,

The chance to learn,
And the chance to play.

No one could keep 373 from falling asleep.
Eyes close silently at 3:13.

I know I'll die before I wake, so please lord, my soul to take.
Brother @@@@
Mother _____.
Father ********
Sister shows up late and now there's nothing she can say.

Wake up!
Wake up! I love you Lil Sis!
Wake up…
Sister _____.

It's an easy scribble
On a sheet of 'scription,
If you're a steady doc
With a good Bic.

But to the mother, the brother, the long-distanced father--just rubble.
Trash left on the beach
far from the transformation back to collectible memories.
Big Sister _____.

Thank you lord for my last day,
You gave me a chance,
Not just to learn, but to play.
Please, guard my family through the night. And keep Big Sister safe till morning's light.
Goodnight.

The Accident

I merge onto the 405, and the fatigue nearly takes me out. I have never felt anything like this before. Not this intensely.

The drive continues, but the exhaustion becomes something I can't control. It's not a fair fight.

All of the sudden, my eyes jolt open. I've accelerated.

What just happened?

I am now two exits past where I was a moment ago. I skipped two exits. Where did I go…unconscious?

There aren't any cars in front of me or to the sides of me. I let out an audible sigh.

I turn the AC higher, max-cold, turn the music up and roll down all the windows.

Again, all the sudden, my eyes open as I'm passing the go-cart racing center.

When did I pass the Goodyear blimp?

I am at least fifteen exits ahead of where I remember being. I haven't even felt the time pass.

BAM!

I hit the car in front of me, throwing my car off balance. It nearly flips as I swerve dramatically the other direction.

SMACK

into the second car on my right.

I swerve again.

Shaking my head, I try to regain my eyesight. My car wobbles and miraculously regains balance.

I just smashed into two cars on the freeway. I just ran into the back of two cars going sixty mph on the freeway!

Does anybody know how to handles this? I have no idea what I'm doing!

I am apathetic. My brain is unresponsive to the circumstances. I do not know how to handle myself. It is like I've forgotten who I am, I've forgotten how to feel.

So I keep driving. I can't figure out how to make my body follow my brain. I am zombie-like as the two damaged cars file off at the next exit. I follow because, thank God, I connect the dots about what had happened and what I need to do.

Just follow them, my subconscious says, and then reiterates; Kali, just follow them.

I park behind the two cars at a gas station, turn around to check if Stella is okay and open my door to face them. I'm numb. I don't even know how to speak.

The two ladies are okay. They are talking at me, but it's as if someone has pressed the mute button along with the quarter-speed button on my world.

Maybe it's shock?

I feel nothing. I come to, realizing that the women are now shouting at me:

"I don't understand," I say, to no one in particular, hoping someone will rescue me from this state of mind.

I hit two cars going sixty on the freeway, and the only reason I pulled off is that I saw them do it. I don't know why I followed them. My Higher Self made the decision for me I guess, brain override.

"What happened?" one of the ladies shouts at me.

I mumble back to her, "I think I fell asleep."

"Fell asleep!? You fell asleep!?" the bigger lady says.

As they ask for my information, I sit, shaking like a leaf, in the front seat of my car. I'm drained and confused.

"Excuse me?" the thin women inquires. She's kindly handing me a notepad and pen. "You are going to want to take down our names, license plates, phone numbers…" She pauses, reassessing the way she's dealing with me. "Would you like me to help you?"

"That whahahaa—oud, by good, yeah, That wouuuh…" I'm having trouble speaking now, massive trouble speaking.

"What happened?" she asks again, looking worried now.

I stammer quietly, "I think I just fell asleep, I have no idea why or—" I'm racking my brain, desperately looking for answers, working with a brain that seems to be malfunctioning.

Noticing my strange demeanor, she offers to call an ambulance. I return all of her health questions back to her like compliments; offering to call her an ambulance, etc. Thank the Lord, except for some neck pain, both women walk away unscathed. One lady tries to get into her back problems but ceases when the kind woman begins asking about my health.

"No, I'm just confused right now. I'm so so so sorry," I say.

I sit in the front seat of my car, perched like a bird, one leg flailing out the door, gaze locked on the hood. My brain is in complete "I have nothing to say to you mode" and downright disapproving disbelief that my mind had decided to turn me into a vegetable. The man inside the Chevron has come out now.

Please don't come talk to me. Please don't come talk to me.

"You okay? Did you get in an accident? Are you sick?" he fires off in a thick accent.

"I'm okay. Thanks. Sorry, I'm leaving," I say.

Dammit.

"No. Please don't drive if you don't feel good. Stay, stay, I'll call an ambulance," he says.

I give up on being polite. My polite-muscle is overused to the point of destruction from the entire sleeping in a closet routine the weekend prior along with being locked in a hot car for seven hours nursing a hangover. I gently shut my door, start up my car and say to myself:

It's only like fifteen minutes; you can do this.

Getting off at the last ramp, I feel the sensation of losing track of time come over me like a curtain. I smack myself in the face, full force, waiting for the light to change.

You are two streets away from your bed, do not lose control now.

Pushing open the green door to my apartment, I unclip Stella, pull off my Ugg boots and fall face-first onto my bed. I turn to the side only after coming very close to suffocating. I'm not sure if I want to die, cry or if I'm hurting. I'm finished.

I fall asleep on top of all my clothing and Stella.

The sweat beading under my hoodie wakes me up. The sun's beating through the window. It must be late afternoon.

OWWW!

My upper back is killing me!

I unintentionally try to pick up my head to greet Stella.

FUCK. Bad Idea.

It feels like I got hit by a bus. I remember the accident, but it seems like a dream still. There isn't any evidence that it even happened, except for the pain in my spine.

Time to go to the doctor.

Getting to Triage

It's dim in here, but midday sabotages my nap by maneuvering around the plastic shade that hangs in front of the window overlooking my Range Rover, which has just caused less damage than it should have, but enough to suffice as life-altering. I stop myself from retracing my thoughts back to the freeway.
Too much!
I shut them off.
The green fern outside is making an anxious sound, flittering against the propped-open window, signifying Santa Ana winds. The space behind my knees is sticky. My eyelids are warm, and the left side of my forehead, directly under my eyebrow is pounding. Most of all, my neck feels completely tense and strained.
But I'm lying down! Relax, you scoundrel!
My neck doesn't respond. I clumsily roll over onto my parka, the zip-tie attaching the lift ticket to the jacket scratches my face, reminding me of the trip, which slightly worsens the pain.
I shift to find a softer place. I sit up slowly but am startled by the intensity of the pain that shoots down the back of my neck.
ZAH!

I grumble to myself, and Stella, I guess, attempting to keep my head steady as I reach for the pile of sweatshirts and clean shirts tossed onto my bed. I shove them in between my knees and roll to the other side.

"GRRRRrrrrrr..." I say.

Stella makes a tired sound and stands up from her curly position. She walks herself in a circle on my comforter to reposition. Her butt's facing me now. My neck spazzes in pain. I roll back over to my back.

Wait, I just got in a car accident, and I keep sleeping. And I have a terrible throbbing headache, some hot eyelid condition and terrible pain in my neck. I should probably go to the ER... Nah, I should go to the doctor... less dramatic.

One...two...three... And I'm up...almost.

I fall back onto my bed letting my legs pop off the ground as I hit. My arms flail out to the sides. I exhale. The familiar Vitruvian Man position. I am used to this "exhausted beyond repair" feeling. It will take at least three days to feel good enough to take Stella for a walk. I knew this feeling. It's not a good one.

Damn it's hot in here.

Still on my back, I scan the room for shoes of any kind. I just need shoes. I go from pile to pile.

My backpack with toiletries is spilled next to the door; an empty prescription bottle is thrown into the chaos. A mostly empty zip-lock bag holds a few pills. A small blue one calls to me. Xanax would probably make this pain more doable. But I am so tired, and with no Adderall left I won't be able to bear the exhausting effects from it enough to make it to the doctor.

The thought of this pulls the last bit of energy out of the depths of me, and I slump down further. I scan the room some more.

My snowboard falls from its post against the dog crate. But my snowboard boots are laced together next to it. Those won't work.

I need damn shoes I can walk in.

The unnecessarily large pile of unsorted ski clothes from the two bags I brought in from the trip is mixed in with the pile of snowboard clothes I had retrieved from Newport before I left for the trip. Everything from bear-head-shaped hats, goggles, gloves, more goggles more glove inserts, hand warmers: everything I could get my hands on from the "ski" box at my parent's house is sprawled out across my studio apartment.

I was in a rush to pack and had decided to bring more than less. I liked the idea of the 'seventies tricolored turtleneck that had once been my dad's, paired with the Koala hat from my childhood. Maybe my mom's white ski pants with the red scarf and the bear hat.

reported.

What Fucking Floor?!

The door clunks shut behind me. My neck feels much stiffer as I realize the difficulty of turning around and locking the door behind me. Flipping through my keychain for the apartment key jerks my head just the slightest and I wince. It is way too bright for this headache. I walk down the emerald green cement steps to the pavement of the driveway.

"UGH!!!" I moan.

Sunglasses on, messy bun flopping, I trudge down Carmelina yet again.

Today it is particularly shameful.

Twenty minutes later I'm in front of the main entrance to the four-story health clinic. Throwing my sunglasses into my purse, I squint at the sign out front.

"What fucking floor?" I say out loud.

In this shape, I could care less who hears me. I need help.

The cold office air washes over me as I enter the building. I'm in no shape to react, so everything just involuntarily tenses up, squeezing a little more pain out of my upper back. Noting my disheveled appearance, I recognize the look in the nurse's eyes as she kindly asks: "Do you have any appointment, sweetheart?"

"No," I say, "But I just got in a car accident. I fell asleep or something on the freeway. I really don't know what's going on."

The nurse is already on my side of the desk, having walked around to usher me forward into triage.

My insides hurt, and my throat clenches. The shame begins to pour out of me onto the chart in front of me. The nurse is scribbling furiously.

"I fell asleep. I blacked out or something. I don't remember. And then, all of the sudden, boom, I felt the jolt before I came back to, well, reality, and I'd hit a car. My car wobbled like a top, or something and momentum was out of my control. I tried to swerve and straighten out, but it was too late. I smacked into a car in the lane on the other side of me. The car leaned so far to each side—" I say.

"And did you stop?" the nurse asks.

"Yeah, but it was weird. I was completely confused about what had happened or what to do. It took me a few moments to wake up. And then I got a message: Just follow the cars off the freeway…" I explain.

I am looking down while explaining the accident, unable to process what occurred. I find it difficult to believe what I am saying. But when I look up, the nurse is standing in front of me, head cocked to one side, and chart folded into her arms.

"You need to go to the emergency room right away," she says. "We will take you over there by ambulance or by wheelchair, you decide."

UC TRIAGE CENTER: APRIL 11, 2011 5:45 PM

TRIAGE VISIT

INITIAL ASSESMENT
REASON FOR VISIT: MVA

SUBJECTIVE
19 y.o. female came to triage at 6pm

reports MVA at 12:25pm today, reports she was driving today and fell asleep at the wheel going 75-80 mph on the freeway. [She] states she hit one car and then tried to steer clear but was unable to avoid hitting 2nd car. Felt out of it, got out of car, states she exchanged information with the drivers. Continued to feel out of it, felt like she was "in shock". Reports she does not recall much of the accident but does recall getting a jolt to the chest with the steering wheel, does not recall the air bag deploying, not sure if she hit her head . no SOB [shortness of breath], no diff[iculty] breathing , body aches, upper back pain, some neck pain, denies head pain, both arms and knees hurt. No officer at the scene.

[She was] able to drive home to sleep and when she woke thought she should come to get evaluated, no appt.s left.

states thinks she was wearing her seatbelt .

denies any alcohol or drugs

ASSESMENT
Motor Vehicle Accident at 12:45 p.m. today

Fell sleep at the wheel

multiple injuries

PLAN
consult with Dr. Douglas, refer to ER - called to inform them she is coming, referral given. DMV form filled

CLINICIAN CONSULTATION NOTES
• Chart note reviewed.

• Discussed clinical presentation, findings, and plan of care with care provider

From Medical Board of California 2010 Guide to Practice of Medicine Page 75, D. Lapses of Consciousness;

All physicians must report immediately in writing to the LHO the name, date of birth, and address of every patient at least 14 years of age or older whom the physician has diagnosed as having a case of a disorder characterized by lapses of consciousness … "Disorders characterized by lapses of consciousness" means those medical conditions that involve:

1. a Loss of consciousness or a marked reduction of alertness or responsiveness to external stimuli; and

2. the inability to perform one or more activities of daily living; and

3. the impairment of the sensory motor functions used to operate a motor vehicle.

Pt. needs to be reported.

EMERGENCY ROOM: APRIL 11, 2011
EMERGENCY ROOM VISIT
ENCOUNTER SUMMARY
OUTCOME: Discharge
FAMILY WAITING: No
LOCATION: Home
CONDITION: Satisfactory
CHIEF COMPLAINT: Back Pain - neck and head. S/P [status post] MVC. [motor vehicle collision. No KO [knockout.]
DIAGNOSIS: Cervical Sprain rx Motrin 400mg 3 x daily, Tylenol 100mg every 4-6 hours, Vicodin
CUSTOM NOTES: you were seen in the ED for multiple complaints following a car accident. You refused any further imaging, CT scan of your brain or neck to rule out potentially serious injury. If you change your mind, are feeling worse, have vomiting, any new neurologic symptoms like weakness, loss of sensation or any other worsening symptoms return to the ED immediately.

DR. BRAUN: APRIL 11, 2011 (EMAIL)
Mode of Contact: Email
FROM: BRAUN, ALEC J. (4/11/2011)4:45:11 PM)
TO: HEALY, KATE
SUBJECT: HI KATE, WONDER

Hi Kate,
Wondered if this student scheduled an appointment with you, which you kindly made available.

DR. HEALY (PHD, PSYCHOLOGIST): APRIL 12, 2011 (EMAIL)

Mode of Contact: Email
FROM: HEALY, KATE (4/12/2011)4:31:16 PM)
TO: BRAUN, ALEC J.
SUBJECT: HI KATE, WONDER

Just saw her for the first time today. She scheduled an additional session for this week.
Thanks,
Kate

FROM: BRAUN, ALEC (4/12/2011) 4:47:09 PM)
TO: HEALY, KATE
SUBJECT: HI KATE, WONDER

Thank you Kate. That is great news!
Signed by Alec Braun, PhD on 4/12/2011 4:48:22 PM
on 4/12/2011 4:48:22 PM

DR. BRAUN: APRIL 12, 2011 (TELEPHONE/EMAIL)

Mode of Contact: Telephone
Follow up for April 7, appt. VM left, call back requested
Mode of Contact: Email
FROM: BRAUN, ALEC
TO: WHEELER, KALI RAE
SUBJECT: I REMAIN HOPEFUL

I remain hopeful that you are doing well.

Today, I wanted to follow-up with you regarding your missed appointment with me on 4/7/11. Prior to, and since your missed appointment, Dr. Kate left voicemail messages with you regarding scheduling. At this time, we have not heard back from you. Please know that I strongly recommend that you schedule a follow-up appointment with me in order to schedule longer term services with unlimited sessions on campus. Per our previous understanding I will go ahead and contact your ongoing provider. Dr. Fiaschetti in order to advise her that you have elected not to pursue services with us if I do not hear from you by Friday. The best times to reach me on weekdays are between 12 - 1pm and 4 - 5pm. On Thursdays, it is best to contact me between 11-12pm.

If you have any questions please do not hesitate to call. And, as always, please recall that we have walk-in appointments between 10am and 4:30 M-F. We also have a ProtoCall Hotline Service available on weekends, holidays and between 5pm and 8am M-F. In case time is emergency, you can always contact the UCPD, 911, or go to the Hospital ER.

Best Wishes,
Alec Braun PhD

DR. DOUGLAS: APRIL 12, 2011
PRIMARY CARE VISIT

INITIAL ASSESMENT

REASON FOR VISIT: MVA

ASSESSMENT

19 yo [year old] Cauc [Caucasian] female … presents following MVA yesterday. Patient reports falling asleep while driving on freeway, striking 2 moving cars. Patient reports R knee and hip pain, neck/back pain, HA, and L shoulder pain. Patient was seen in RR Hosp and was diagnosed with cervical sprain. A CT scan and cervical films were reportedly recommended, but patient left without undergoing these studies. Patient denies alcohol or drug use prior to incident. No scalp or facial pain. Patient with central chest discomfort, worse with deep breath or with palpation of chest wall. Neck pain is predominantly posterior, and worse with movement. Patient with upper back and interscapular pain, as well as milder low back pain. Patient reports superficial abdominal pain, worse with palpation or tensing of abdominal musculature. Patient notes decreased ability to concentrate. Memory is normal, though patient only recalls some details of accident.

DEVICES GIVEN: Cervical Collar 5:51 p.m.

PLAN

Rec [recommended] X-rays and further evaluation now in ER [emergency room.] Patient declines [the ER trip], understanding that spinal point tenderness may be associated with vertebral fracture, and that delay in evaluation of an unstable fracture may result in permanent paralysis, disability, or death. Patient refuses transfer to ER. She verbalizes her understanding of discussion, and accepts the risk of non-compliance with my best medical opinion.

Rest. Avoid aggravating activities. Cervical collar for comfort. RTC [return to clinic] tomorrow for X-rays and re-evaluation.

RADIOLOGY: APRIL 13, 2011
RADIOLOGICAL REPORT
ORDERED BY: Douglas, Matthew M.D.
19 yo female S/P MVA with neck and upper back pain, worse at approx T3.
IMPRESSION
No plain radiographic evidence for acute cervical or thoracic spine finding.

DR. DOUGLAS: APRIL 13, 2011
PRIMARY CARE VISIT

INITIAL ASSESMENT
REASON FOR VISIT: F/U MVA
Patient returns for F/U MVA. Patient is still somewhat confused by incident, but reports being drowsy before lapse in alertness. Patient was able to answer questions immediately after accident. No tongue bite or incontinence. No h/o seizure. Notes improved, but persistent HA. Neck pain is better with use of cervical collar. Interscapular pain is moderate to occ severe in intensity, worse with deep breath. No SOB, fever/chills, NN. No true muscle weakness. Patient reports h/o extremity numbness/tingling. No change since accident. Chest wall tenderness is better, but ribs are still sore. Patient reports decreased abdominal muscle pain. No bruising. Hip is better. Patient took 2 Vicodin yesterday evening and one this morning. Patient will see psychiatrist tomorrow.
Patient reports an episode one day prior to accident in which friends told patient that she was awake, but unresponsive, for approx 15 minutes.
Patient also reports h/o slow and rapid pulse, occ associated with lightheadedness.

ASSESSMENT
RADIOLOGY RESULTS: Kyphoscoliosis
DIAGNOSIS:
S/P MOTOR VEHICLE ACCIDENT
HEADACHE
PALPITATIONS

PLAN
X-ray reviewed. Will prescribe Flexeril as need for Vicodin decreases. Referral to PT. RTC [return to clinic] 1 week, sooner or to ER for worsening. Report to DMV [department of motor vehicles] already submitted. Referral to Neurology. Obtain EKG (patient declines now, but will RTC for study). Referral to Cardiology. NO DRIVING or other activities that may expose patient to risk should she experience a lapse in consciousness.

VERIFICATION OF ILLNESS
This note is being requested by the above patient to verify medical illness or fitness after illness for academic/administrative/employment purposes.
probable duration of disability: 1 week
Disability and absence from class due to injuries sustained in automobile accident.
Signed Andrew Douglas M.D.

BELLE HOFFMAN (WHNP): APRIL 15, 2011
WOMEN'S HEALTH VISIT
INITIAL ASSESSMENT
REASON FOR VISIT: Annual
ASSESMENT/PLAN

D/C NuvaRing now--I removed it for pt. [patient], to make appt. in neuro[logy] ASAP., to cont. with BHI. F/U with PCP [primary care physician], Dr. Douglas M.D.

ANDREA NGUYEN (M.D., CARDIOLOGIST): APRIL 18, 2011

CARDIOLOGY

REASON FOR CONSULTATION
Presyncope and syncope.

HISTORY OF PRESENT ILLNESS:
Ms. Wheeler is a 19-year-old female who has a long history of dizziness as well as possible syncopal episodes. She describes these syncopal episodes as moments where there is a lapse of consciousness and not aware of her surroundings, although it appears her eyes are open during these episodes. She was recently involved in a motor vehicle accident on the freeway, where she rear-ended another person. She is unsure at this time if this episode was associated with a loss of consciousness. She also describes at this time chronic chest pain at rest as well as with activity, usually around the ribs, as well as chronic dyspnea and chronic palpitations, usually with exercise. She routinely runs up to 2 miles as well as dances, and notes slight increase in chest pain as well as dyspnea during these activities. She denies any symptoms of heart failure including orthopnea, PND, or lower extremity edema.

PHYSICAL EXAMINATION
Vital signs: General: Well-developed, well-nourished young female appearing stated age, in no acute distress. Cardiovascular: Regular rate and rhythm. Neurologic: No focal weakness. Sensation intact to light touch. Psychiatric: Alert and oriented. Normal mood and affect.

IMPRESSION
1. Presyncope and possible syncope. Appears less likely to be of cardiac etiology or history, however, cannot exclude.

2. Chest pain, atypical for ischemia. 3. Palpitations. 4. Bipolar disorder. 5. Hypothyroid. 6. Attention deficit disorder. 7. Chronic fatigue syndrome.

RECOMMENDATIONS
1. Check transthoracic echocardiogram to evaluate for any structural heart disease.

2. Check Holter monitor for any arrhythmia.

3. Check an exercise treadmill test for any exercise-induced arrhythmia.

4. Recommend to check baseline labs including CBC, comprehensive metabolic panel, TSH per PMD.

5. Consider, check HIV.

6. I will see the patient back within 2 weeks after the aforementioned studies have been performed.

7. Check pulmonary function testing.

Thank you for allowing me to participate in the care of this patient. Please feel free to contact me with any additional questions. Signed Andrea Nguyen, M.D.

DOUGLAS, ANDREW, (M.D.): APRIL 20, 2011
PRIMARY CARE VISIT

INITIAL ASSESSMENT
REASON FOR VISIT: F/U after MVA

SUBJECTIVE
Patient returns with improvement in musculoskeletal symptoms, but HAs have continued (without increase). Patient continues with daily HA, moderate in intensity and rarely severe. Neck and interscapular > low back pain. No signif[icant] chest discomfort or abdominal pain felt by patient to be related to accident. Patient reports difficulty with concentration and mild problems with memory, as well as an "out or it" or cloudy thinking sensation.

ASSESSMENT
DIAGNOSIS:
POST-CONCUSSION SYNDROME
  NECK PAIN
  BACK PAIN

PLAN:
Continue acetaminophen prn and naproxen bid [BY MOUTH] with food. F/U cardiology, neurology, and PT. No driving (patient denies driving). RTC 1-2 weeks, sooner for worsening.

LINDSAY AGUILLON, (N.P.): APRIL 20, 2011
CHART MEMO

Faxed morbidity report—episodes of "black outs" syncope—to 888-xxx-xxx
informed patient this report was sent
called patient now, states she is feeling better, has appts with cardiology and Dr. Douglas, understands she cannot drive until resolved

DR. DOUGLAS: APRIL 21, 2011
Referral to outside specialist: Dr. Olivera (neurology)
DIAGNOSIS:
Post-concussion syndrome
Petit mal epilepsy

A Poem for Dr. Braun: April 23, 2011

Circling phrases from a nicely printed flyer:
"Boosting Test Performance,"
"Keys to a happy relationship,"
"Psychology of happiness," falling on the same day as
"Healthy Ways of Dealing With Stress," and "Staying Motivated," comes next in a different room on the next day.

So many keys
Which one will open the door
And is that door meant to be opened
Should that door stay shut
Why listen to you
I bet your marriage isn't great
I can smell the tobacco on your nicely flattened kakis, Love.

My favorite thing
To ask how you are feeling today
Locked up in your small room
Listening to disgruntled college students
Yearning for something you can't give them

I try not to talk too sadly
I don't want to upset your fragile state, doctor
It's okay we don't have to talk about it
I wouldn't want to prod into your home-life
It's just the reason why I am being so difficult

I don't want to make you cry.

A Friendly Neurologist

I go to a neurologist to figure out what happened the day of my accident. I tell doctors everything. I feel like they need to know every last detail about me to make the correct diagnosis. For instance, on intake forms, those rows of boxes that that say:

"Have you had, do you have, or have you ever had any of the following symptoms/conditions" followed by rows of answers, "never," "sometimes," "always."

Those forms and all those options are my worst nightmare. I am thorough, to say the least. I go through each box and think about it thoroughly before checking a box and moving onto the next box. There are ten full pages boxes and questions. I go through each one.

The question in it of itself doesn't make grammatical, or even, logical sense. But, I fill it out to the best of my ability. I should have known better. I've always had an issue with telling too much of the story, being too honest.

After a short wait, a young, casual-seeming Dr. Olivera strolls in flipping through my chart. "You're so young to be having so much going on! Let's figure this out." He looks up at me smiling.

"You can try…" I say.

Do you know how many doctors have told me that, sir?

"Why do you say that?" he asks.

"Because no one can ever figure me out," I say.

"We will see about that," he says.

He touches a couple tender spots on the back of my head. He has me take a vision test, follow his finger in different directions, say the alphabet forward and backwards (which is already hard for me I have to sing from like "g" on). He does strength tests and asks me to hold my arms out straight while he scans me from the far wall of the room. We do a verbal memory test as well as a verbal math-problem sequence, and then he puts his clipboard down.

"I see you didn't check a box under 'using alcohol,'" the doctor says.

"Yeah, I used to drink a lot and now not at all," I say.

"A lot quantity-wise in one sitting or a lot meaning often?" he asks.

"A lot like I can handle way more than I should be able to. I'm pretty small and can drink anyone under the table and seem sober, but my memory completely turns itself off. It's like I have a tipping point..." I explain.

"And you wrote you were in a program. Is it a 12-step program?" he says.

"Yeah, I try to get to meetings, but to be honest, it doesn't really fit my case," I say.

"Were you drinking prior to the accident?" he asks.

"What? Of course not, I don't do that," I say.

"Did you take anything?" he asks.

"No," I say.

"You told the nurse at triage you had just been on a trip," he says.

"Yeah with the Snowboarding Club," I say.

"Did you drink while on the trip?" he asks.

I stutter for a moment, wondering why that would matter. "Yeah," I say.

"So you drank before this happened, in the days prior to your accident?" he asks.

"Yeah but—" I say.

"Kali, look at me," he walks up close to me, my feet dangling off of the sterile white paper covering of the exam table. His eyes are vivid blue, almost unnaturally so, but they are transfixing. I try not to smirk, but he's so close to me, I become shy, which is very rare. It almost feels as if he'll fall into me at any moment, but his arms are crossed tightly over the clipboard on his chest. "Look at me." The doctor unfolds his arms, "You need to get into a program for alcoholics. Go to your meetings and focus on staying sober. It works if you work it..."

"Work it cause you're worth it," I recite with him.

I finally understand where he is coming from. There's a moment of silence as I recognize him as a partner in this, someone to confide in. But this is the exact moment where I get it wrong. Just because it is obvious to me he is a recovering addict, it doesn't mean that he wants to share that information with me. Or that I should trust him.

I should have the not-trusting part down, but I somehow can't shake the overly trusting part of myself. I want to know more about him and the way to do that, is to spill about myself.

Worst. Idea. Ever.

I pull out my car-keys to show him my serenity prayer keychain.

"Well, you won't be needing those," the doctor says.

"Huh?" I say.

"You are not legally allowed to drive anymore," he says.

"Wait, what? Why?" I say.

"Relax, it's protocol. You reported a loss of consciousness at the emergency room. They are required to send that information to the DMV, who will send you an official notice of revocation in the mail," he says.

"What? What about my car? And my life! And work!" I almost shout.

"Here's a tip: They will probably take a couple weeks to sort through the paperwork. You can legally drive until you get the notice. However, if you do drive with a suspended license, after you receive the notice, along with the accident you got into, they will take your license forever. They are very strict with this rule. So once you get that notice, do not drive."

In disbelief, tears well up under my eyelids. I fumble with the now childish keychain I wanted him to admire.

He says, "I'm going to order up a brain scan, and set up an appointment for you to see the cardiologist. It may have had to do with your heart not pumping correctly. And I see here that you have a T-wave abnormality." He flips a piece of paper and continues. "Also, I need you to report back to me a completely sober couple of weeks until our next visit. I am going to give you a medicine for pain and to replace the Depakote you had been taking prior to the accident. It's called Savella. It should help you tremendously. Do you have any questions for me?"

He looks up coldly.

"No," I say. I'm shocked by the change in his demeanor and he notices. He holds his hand out for a handshake.

"Be good. Don't drink. Don't drive. And promise me you will be safe with the people you surround yourself with," the doctor says. He releases my hand and walks away. He stops in the doorway. "I get the impression that you allow too many people around you. Trust is to be earned, Kali."

"Thanks," I say.

OLIVERA, KYLE (M.D., NEUROLOGIST) : APRIL 25, 2011
REASON FOR VISIT: Referral
REFERRING DOCTOR: Andrew Douglas M.D.
A/P: Ordered CAT scan.
Rx Savella (See Appendix T.)

Mistress Overcome: Spring 2011

Mistress waits for the Stella Artois,
To slide across the Lonestar distance,
She's pretty,
a picture,
a gem,
a flower.
She sings to herself of the wandering hour.
So, I'm gonna smile…
She repeats and the song concludes,
Because I want to see you happy,
…laugh…
Stiff,
rigid,
perfect—
the seamlessly conducted orchestra of hers falls out of sync.
The shell of Mistress Overcome splintered,
causes a cameraman to be stolen from his picture.
And so a lens captures a new angle,
a recherché frame,
Mistress commonly keeps this side of her contained
Dark amber juices,
and clear viscous liquids
contrast with walls of long-lost days,
when longing had its place and time.
It overflows the banks—
and crushes the flood gates built up so exceptionally-well—
like every device in her arsenal
of latches, clasps and locks.
Long-awaited laughter,
Won't even show its reflection.
She waits for an echo…
none to expose.

Hold it together, Mistress! Smile, Beautiful, it's time to take your picture!

And she will.
But tonight the external cannot fight its other.
Her makeup fades away
to reveal an ounce of her ten-ton pain.
Deep set eyes,

and honeycomb locks reveal a stolen smile--
her joy creases faded
along with her sense of the real versus the sublime.
Fallen into the void
along she goes for the ride.
Wishful thoughts to decipher the equation,
how to turn the arms of his back equal.
Erase—
What's gone a Miss-
tres?
Empty—
She's left in a snow-globe.

Sparkling glimpses,
like this one stay true,
to the documentation
of the watering lashes
of Mistress Overcome,
yet to be known as
Mistress Overcame.
Take it away Zinfandel.
Take cover, Mistress.
Take care, let it take over.
Mistress Overcome has been left for the lesser.
    Sometimes the spirits should last a couple minutes longer.

Interlude: All My Friends Are Doctors

With all of these doctors, I felt like I could show them something. I wanted them to know everything about me for a reason. I might not have known the exact reason at the time, but I wanted to show them that I wasn't well. I always wanted to show them that. I wanted to show them that I wasn't well and that I wasn't common. I wanted them to know that I was different. I was different. But that they were capable doctors who could help me by just allowing my body to help itself.

If I spilled my guts to the doctors, they would then be able to put me back together.

However, instead of putting me back together, they would tear me apart.

Drugged by the DJ...for My Birthday

I have knack when it comes to concerts and getting backstage passes. I've never done anything groupie-like, but in my drunken escapades, I've seemed to sense things. For example, I think the two middle-aged folks behind me are the keyboardist's parents. And then, saying to myself, why the fuck not, I turn around, mid-song, to compliment them on their son.

We then have a sincere conversation, which wouldn't have gone as nicely if they hadn't been his parents. Along with the shocked look on his face, (that his conservative parents have brought along a young girl), the guy rips off his "All Access" badge and tells me to go for it.

"I don't know what it's good for, but try it out. I know Ellie Goulding is back there if you like her..."

It is always easy to find one seat open. Then I have to negotiate with the people next to me (i.e., scoot super close to them, smile, and then drag my friend into the space I have been inhabiting). If there is a guy with me, it is usually a problem. I've never cared enough about any of the guys I dated to fight for their space, so I tuck them in close behind or wave at them to come one up here, knowing that the journey is pretty much impossible.

Tonight is an accurate example of my ability to accidently run into the talent.

Gatsby is back in LA after another stint in rehab. He now owns a home with Elijah (remember him) in the most luxurious neighborhood in our town, Newport Coast. I'm not sure what they do all day, but Elijah now owns a clothing line that is promoted by the likes of basically every professional athlete who is into fashion, from basketball to football, the guy has managed to charter private jets, attend their birthday parties and get them to wear a piece of the line in a million photos. Not too bad for a guy who got in trouble for pistol whipping someone in the rival gang from the opposite side of the bay, with a very expensive handgun.

I drive alone to the highly regarded night club. I am meeting Jaxx there, and I feel I have been hanging out with him as a friend long enough. I invite JJ along, just for kicks. I don't think he'll show.

JJ is the audio engineer and producer of a band I meet after Mikah and I split. We met at their debut music video shoot a couple weeks. He is shy, but he takes a cute picture of me and allows me to ask him a ton of questions about audio engineering when he leaves the shoot to grab cigarettes at the local store.

He owns a construction business up the coast and is building a recording studio currently in a warehouse not far from his job about an hour up the coast from Los Angeles. His drive is fascinating, as well as his ability to literally build this warehouse into a studio from the ground up.

JJ is living on the weekdays at a home in Hollywood that years ago functioned as a major recording. He is building his own recording studio in Santa Barbara, from the ground up, while still working for the family construction business and attending a top-notch audio engineering school (that I would become very enamored with).

JJ invited me to Santa Barbara with Stella to hang, wrap cables, record a bit and promote the bands that were recording there. I began spending weekends at the Santa Barbara studio, he built a one bedroom place above the studio with a shower and everything. I brought my dog, leather journal, homework and guitar and JJ showed me the meaning of making your dreams come true. JJ recently fled a religion that acted like a cult, so I celebrated his first birthday with him.

He lets me crash at the Hollywood studio the night we meet.

To my surprise, JJ shows up at the club. And, he has to pay for a table and a bottle before being let in. Awkward would be the wrong word for this. It is cringe-worthy to watch JJ, ten years Jaxx's senior, finally get let into the club an hour after arriving, and then meet Jaxx and me lounging comfortably on the VIP sofas.

I am embarrassed.

"Hey! So glad you could come," I say.

"Yah, they made me buy a bottle," JJ says.

"Sucks, bro," Jaxx says carelessly and shouts to his diamond-studded buddy.

"Yo, Jaxx, come get some of this," one of Jaxx's friends calls over to him. The guy is impeccably dressed. He looks like Jaxx to me: that familiar, clean look that I grew up around. I immediately feel a tinge of embarrassment as I catch a glimpse of JJ's beat-up Vans and I take a sip of the vodka Cranberry I'm holding and re-cross my legs to face him.

It isn't long before I hear a familiar voice.

"Oh my God! It's Malik Arnette!"

Malik Arnette is a hugely popular Def Jam RnB singer that I loved. Not only did I love singing along to his songs, I danced to his music on the competition teams all my life.

I scan the crowded club to find Jaxx. He's staring back at me from the pool area. He motions for me to come to him. He's lying on what looks like a ginormous beanbag while acrobats twist and turn, practically naked, above the rectangular pool running through the lounge area.

He has done this for me.

Without a word, I slip away to meet Gatsby and fall into the beanbag where he's lying.

"Thank you," I say quietly looking at him.

He says nothing as I lie there in ecstasy next to him, wishing we could go back to where we once were.

"Anytime," Jaxx finally responds.

The loud club goes silent and we lie together for a minute. I love being with him. He calms me down. He keeps me safe.

"Go up there! Go have fun," Jaxx says.

I don't move, soaking in the serenity of the moment with Jaxx.

"Where?" I ask.

"You love Malik Scott, right? And it looks like he loves you too. He's totally staring at you," Jaxx says.

"You didn't!" I shout.

I look at the stage and sure enough Malik Scott keeps looking over at me.

I make my way through the drunk mess of people and finally get to the stage.

"Grab my hand," Malik Scott says, his arm-outstretched, ready to lift me onto the stage.

Is he really looking at me right now?! This has to be a dream.

Without a word, I'm easily lifted onto the stage. He swings his arm around my waist. I think two things: 1) Jaxx is the best and is probably really happy to see this and 2) JJ probably left after seeing this.

The difference between the two reactions is enough to make me decide I never want to hang with JJ again. Jaxx reminds me what it feels like to be loved. He always did that, even when he didn't mean to.

Looking down at my watch, I see it's 1:00 a.m.

"It's my Birthday!" I say quietly.

The DJ starts up the next track. The singer says, into the mic, like a true showman, "If today is your birthday, baby girl, this surely has to be fate."

As he sings, it gets a bit crowded by the front of the stage where he's been using me as a puppet. Wanting to escape the awkwardness of feeling like I'm about to fall into the crowd below every time he moves an inch, I scoot myself out from under his arm and manage to get behind him. I'm leaning against the DJ booth after tripping over a couple mic cables.

The DJ shouts, one ear out of his headphones: "Drink this! Happy birthday!"

He pulls out a jumbo-sized bottle of very expensive champagne.

"You sure?" I ask, not wanting to drink thousands of dollars of their champagne.

He looks at me and nods, "Positive." He's still manipulating the turntables all the while.

After a couple swigs, he does a "cut off" motion with his hand like a salute, but lower. He motions for me to hand the bottle back to him, motioning again for me to lean into him.

"No more baby girl. That's enough," the DJ says.

Black.

I don't remember a moment more of that night.

Mr. Wrong: Spring 2011

Intoxicated exclamations overshadow the near-eatable moon tonight. Slurred, sloppy conversations, unsuccessful exchanges and a multitude of matching little black dresses lay out the backdrop of Act I tonight. Oversized women smushed into attractive shapes with leather and lace, parade themselves through the obstacles, clutching glasses to their hearts, a welcome sign for Mr. Right. Someday the sign won't have to ignite. But they wait…

Mr. Wrongs walk in 3 X 3—sardines releasing pheromones hungry for estrogen, smooth legs and all the rest. They're starving for a dressing room to slip on the latest perfume, and the Wrongs progress to Rights as the night swirls on. Pass the tonic and gin and let DJ Krude spin them all into a state of oblivion.

Mr. Right catches Mike—ear bud intact, stone-faced, holding the guest list—an idyllic figure it seems—or perhaps to some a guarantor of finding Mrs. Right. But tonight the unresolved issues of the child in Mikah destine him to be a bit uptight and Mr. Right is denied entry. He falls victim to the blaring lamps and boastful streetlights, expressing his loneliness with a sigh and a song. And so it goes, streetlight people…
He makes his Journey home.
The North star winks.
Coincidentally…

Mrs. Right hurries amidst the decadent glow. Luna reveals her solemn face. A long workday leads to a sense of fulfillment, but she knows she'll sleep alone again tonight.

The youngest whines a few streets up. Shivering alongside her big brother, beneath the moon glow and reflections of moonshine bottles echoing from the kitchen window, they do as Mother told them to: Look to the moon. And so they do. Whenever I am gone, wherever I may be, look to the sky at night and I'll be right by your side.

To the two jewels of Mrs. Right this is a song of melancholy and longing to be held by mommy. Tonight's the night to sing to Luna, Big Brother and Little Sister need to escape the void of the lonely universe. Mommy, please come home.

Mrs. Right lingers on, reminiscing on easy mornings with Mr. Wrong, who just happened to feel so right, at the time. She knows that somewhere out there, Mr. Right yearns to sing along with her. And so it goes, some will win, some will lose ... She falls asleep staring up at a torn picture in a broken frame. It goes on and on and on...

Moving & Paint Therapy

The day comes to move into my new Carmelina apartment and having broken up with Mikah recently, I have to move my stuff alone. I end up manually carting my moving boxes in one of the rolling move-in carts from the dorms. They litter the sidewalks during move-in week.

The new place is only two blocks up on Carmelina Ave. However, right at the top of the steep driveway up from the old apartment, the sidewalk takes another steep incline up the hill.

Alone and crazy on Savella, I push my mess of belongings, thrown in the Dumpster-shaped crate, backward up the cracked driveway.

The first Carmelina apartment is being torn down after I reported a cockroach problem to my landlord, swearing to him I am not a slob. He reveals the news that the entire building is being torn down by the end of the month, due to that problem.

So, in fact, the one (or maybe three) times I left Domino's pizza boxes on the table in the kitchen didn't cause the cockroaches to swarm.

I cockroach-bomb the place so many times that I feel my things, along with a partial section of my lungs, are covered in the toxic spray. I spend hours and hours taping up my belongings to do the feared bomb, and it doesn't even work. I rip off my clothing if I see a roach two rooms away, immediately jumping in the shower.

I even sleep with the light on every night and sound like a murder-victim about seven times a day. Maybe that's why the fraternity next door never bothered me after that one night...

As everyone in my building is moving out, the construction team moves in. The apartments are in the early stages of being demolished the day after the mandatory move-out. Ashlyn, Felix, Jeremih, all of us have to be separated.

My parents come up the next day to help get the new apartment together. I am so overwhelmed the day after the move that I think I am having a seizure. I can't get my words out in the right order. I stutter, then blank-out. My mouth feels like jelly, and my heart is beating so fast, it's visible.

I try to tell my father where I'd like a picture hung, but all of the walls are caving in. My field of vision is getting tiny and I can't tell anyone what is going on because I can't form sentences.

Christina and Felix recognize the expression on my face and know that I need to get outside.

Felix thinks it will be helpful to paint. Megan is an art history major and very talented painter. Felix has kept her painting supplies from when they dated.

Christina agrees, "Yeah, maybe if you focus on the colors—"

"What's going on? Why is she—" my dad asks.

"I don't know," Christina responds, "But Kali seems to respond well when you get stress out of the equation."

"I think it's her medication," Felix says.

"What medication?" my dad asks.

"The one the neurologist gave her. She told me one night that all of a sudden she gets dizzy and she can't form sentences. I've seen it happen. She stutters and her heart races. You can feel it. It's wild," Felix says.

"Okay. If you guys want to take a break, we will finish here," my mom says.

I leave my parents in the pint-sized apartment, along with my scattered boxes and random pilrs of things. We head to Felix's.

Felix has a great two-bedroom place on the third floor in the closest unit to the street. It overlooks the street and is above the chaos. You can see the school from his window, in all of its foliage and brick-accented glory.

It is paint-therapy for me and I immediately start feeling better. I paint huge wings across the entire back wall of the apartment.

Christina, in her usual genius, paints the most sophisticated scenes of flowing thick lines that morph into full-on humans. Felix takes a more-detailed approach, hence the engineering post-graduate degree, and draws geometric designs. The colors vary so drastically between the rooms that it is like an exhibit.

Mark's roommate's room gets the left-over paint-balls. We splash the white walls with a fury of color, having the time of our lives aggressively throwing paintballs at a blank wall of the now deserted third-story apartment that first week of June. It is bliss.

Stella comes with me later that night to explore the space we created, and it is magical.

Angel: Spring 2011

When it's asymmetrical
It's…
When it's unfaltering
It's…
When it's too hazy to discern
It's…
When it's impermeable and still breaking
It's…
All her fault.
No.
Someone took the blame. No.
Someone stole her name.
Angel.
That's it!
Mamma calls her this.
Yet she cannot fulfill the grandeur of Angel,
Not anymore.

I'll just speak to Papa from now on.

Papa can never decipher her voice from her sister's,
When she calls longing for a listen.
In this,
she will escape her name.
But who now is Angel
To blame?

I am to blame. He told me so.

A slurred, porridge of words
left her below a dreaming tree—
dim-lit by neighborhood-watch
lights!
Empty lightning strikes across
a lowly, thunder-struck road,
and Angel gasps for truth.

It's not raining, He told me so!
Acid rain droplets
seep deep into pores

left gaping wide—
gruesome holes—
too willing to house his nonsensical reality,
that Angel began to call home.

Transparency is opaque
under droplets of water,
carefully crafted to appear dry—
Droplets of the sun's rays! he used to exclaim.

Think up an essay Little One.
Mamma says Your star is fading.
And you're her Angel!
You're the one!

He caused a caesura in Angel.
An equilateral morphed obtuse in her eyes,
that found white in black-out conditions
and mowed down warning signs
despite mother's warnings.

Mamma watched Angel's stem snapped,
and crackled,
under the weight of a
sickening, soul-snatching figure—
a sunflower's killer—
just too bright,
just too much light,
Blinded, Angel crashed into his poppy field.
Angel died alongside diabolical footprints of filth-smeared intent.

DR. OLIVERA: MAY 02, 2011
RADIOLOGICAL DIAGNOSTIC REPORT
SIGNS AND SYMPTOMS: POSSIBLE SEIZURES
REQUESTING PHYSICIAN: OLIVERA, KYLE J. M.D.
MR The Brain Epilepsy Protocol
FINDINGS: The cerebral sulci, ventricles and basal cisterns are normal in size and shape. The signal intensity of the brain demonstrates no apparent asymmetry or abnormality. The volumetric sequence shows no evidence of a cortical dysplasia, heterotopic gray matter, or other migration anomaly. The T2 and FLAIR sequences show no signal abnormalities within the cerebrum, brain stem or cerebellum. No evidence of intracranial bleeding is identified and no mass, mass-effect midline shift is seen. No extra-axial fluid collections are noted. The brainstem and cerebellum show no focal lesions. Flow-voids are identified in the large intracranial arteries and dural sinuses, suggesting patency. The visualized paranasal sinuses and mastoid air cells are clear.

IMPRESSION:
This MR of the brain with epilepsy and protocol shows no definite structural abnormalities.

DR. FIASCHETTI: MAY 05, 2011
Geodon♯ (See Appendix O.)

♯ This was the second time she prescribed me Geodon. The first time I hated it was in high school.

DR. OLIVERA: MAY 18, 2011
Department/Specialty: NEUROLOGY

Kali, a 20-year-old female referred in because of lapse in consciousness, resulting in an automobile accident.

The day before coming back from Mammoth Mountain, she had an episode of a lapse in consciousness while sitting in her car. She reports frequent episodes of transient lapses in consciousness of several years' duration. She also admits to blacking out if she drinks heavily.

Two weeks prior to my consult on approximately April 11, or thereabouts on a Monday driving from LA to Newport to pick up her dog. The trip went fine. On the way back, however, she blacked out and hit 2 cars. She was not injured, she traded insurance and license information, and then drove back to Los Angeles. On her return, she took a nap after which she went to a triage nurse at the University center who sent her to the Emergency Room. She saw a doctor there who recommended scans, but she apparently signed out against medical advice.

At the time of the auto accident she cannot remember if she hit her head, and she does not think that she lost consciousness.

In addition to the above problems, she has a history of fibromyalgia and was treated with Neurontin 1000 to 1200 mg tablets a day. (See Appendix I.) Her fibromyalgia was manifested by generalized muscle aches and pains with pain in the neck and back and polyarthralgia. She additionally has a history of psychiatric problems and sees a Dr. Fiaschetti for bipolar disorder and is on Depakote 250 mg a day, which she stopped taking before the trip to Mammoth. (See Appendix Q.) She did use NuvaRing for birth control, which she removed as she was concerned about the possibility of stroke symptoms secondary to this manifested by numbness in her legs and tingling in her hands. [The OBGYN removed this four days after the incident because she was worried about the possibility that NuvaRing had caused a stroke.] (See Appendix S .)

RECOMMENDATIONS:

Suggest MRI scan of the brain with and without contrast and an EEG. The patient will be seen following these studies in reevaluation.

Therapeutically, the patient was started on a 2-week starter pack of Savella for her fibromyalgia with a follow up appointment scheduled. Depending on the results of the EEG, further recommendations regarding the periodic loss of consciousness will follow.

Fan-Mail Repetition

Noble
Upon the woven threads sat the mailman's employers—neatly stacked dominoes of lovely different personalities and styles of handwriting—the praises for my elegant performances and such. An elaborately looked-after envelope appealed to me. It donned a subtle watercolor landscape. Its elegance alerted me to unseal the tongue-induced adhesive. A wonderful surprise! A stone-colored figurine, perfect for the mantle. It made an awful ruckus chipping against the others as I nestled it neatly into my back pocket. It was one of the spectacles that I would rather keep closer to my heart than to the candlesticks oN the mantle.

Word Composition
My mind skedaddled like tasting the rainbow with low blood-sugar, fiending for a drug. Pour some on me! In a uniformed pile of overnighted and American-flagged right corners, my eyes auto tune toward the uninhibited piñata of the bunch. Inside hid an elephant—an orphan, there was just one. Scrumdidiliumpscious! It clinked and clanged and chimed its greeting to the others in my treasure-check pocket.

Ignorant
Rustling through my heaping mound of unopened fan mail, I came across a letter that stuck out from the rest. Though I never really read the letters, when there is a pretty stamp or something like that, I enjoy perusing the inevitably colorful contents within. What a surprise! I didn't know that a toy elephant was the "in" gift at the moment. But it'll do. Anyway, I know it's odd, but I cherish the little things or however that cliché goes…possibly… smelling the roses would work better there? Stop and smell the roses? Whatever. It makes quite an awful amount of noise—maybe clamor is a better word—when it hits up against the other specials I don't pay too much attention to while they're hidden within my back pocket. But, I know they are there, most of the time.

The Vibes Changed

During the next Dr. Olivera appointment, I search for what I saw at that first appointment, where I felt we'd connected, that we were one and the same. Instead, I receive normal results from the brain scan and a date that I can schedule my DMV appointment hearing, if I stay on track (meaning no drinking, no driving.)

Instead of explaining what happened on the freeway that morning, Dr. Olivera focuses all his time on preaching to me about drinking. This is unnecessary, since I already promised myself a while back that I won't be drinking until things are sorted out, and maybe even then, I'll refrain.

I am loving Savella, but he never once asks me about it. He ups my dosage, tells me I seem a lot better and asks if I'd like to try Lyrica for the fibromyalgia. My chart points out that I declined due to previous problems while taking the Lyrica prescribed by Morano; he doesn't seem to notice that.

Before he leaves the room, he stands as close as did at the first appointment, puts his hand on top of mine in my lap and tells me that he believes in me. Without shifting his stance, he continues, emphasizing his point with a gentle squeeze of my hands.

"You are a beautiful, intelligent girl with such a bright future ahead of you. You should be around people who care about you who are not intimidated into using you."

I want to connect with him so badly. I really feel like he will get it. But the last visit is just that, a doctor's visit, and it leaves me cold inside.

I exit the office with nothing gained: no license, no strategy to move forward, and worst, no answers regarding what caused me to blackout on the freeway.

All that Dr. Olivera mentions is a mini-stroke-like pattern. He doesn't confirm anything or say anything further on what seemed to me like a name he has crafted from the symptoms I reported.

DR. OLIVERA: JUNE 14, 2011
Department/Specialty: NEUROLOGY

OUTPATIENT NEUROLOGIC FOLLOWUP

Kali is a 20-year-old, soon to be senior student here, whom I saw initially in consultation on April 24, because of lapse in consciousness resulting in an automobile accident. The patient at that time, reported a long history of psychiatric problems with bipolar disorder, ADHD, as well as binge drinking, which was accompanied at times by alterations in consciousness. The patient additionally has history of fibromyalgia and was treated in the past with Neurontin up to 1200 mg a day, which was not effective. When I first saw her, we ordered an EEG which was negative. An MRI scan, which was negative and some lab which has not yet returned. I have also started her on Savella which she is tolerating quite well, it has alleviated her headaches, her generalized body aches and pains. She states that she has not had anything to drink since April nor has she had any lapses in consciousness, and she denies use of any drugs. She continues under the care of her psychiatrist Dr. Fiaschetti.

PHYSICAL EXAM
Today, Head and neck: Unremarkable. There was minimal tenderness in the cervical paraspinous region but much less so than previously. Vital signs: Blood pressure was 114/70 and pulse was 78. Cardiac: Normal size heart with no murmurs. Neurological: Normal.

IMPRESSION
1. Fibromyalgia with headaches and body aches and pains, responding to Savella.
2. Past history of syncopal spells some related to alcohol and/or drugs, currently asymptomatic.

PLAN
Continue Savella and follow the patient every 6 weeks over the summer. (See Appendix T.)

A Starter Pack to Hell: Savella

The neurologist decides that since everything he tried (a brain scan, radiologist, echogram, as well as a thorough verbal and physical examination) brought about no conclusive results, the reason for my "the lapse of consciousness" is my quick discontinuation of Depakote. (See Appendix Q.) Note that a lapse of consciousness is a general term Dr. Olivera loved using, that can indicate anything from a grand mal seizure to a heart attack, to simply falling asleep.

In its place, he's given me a hearty bag full of sample packs of a new drug, Savella. This drug is supposed to help with that nasty case of fibromyalgia he noted in his records. The problem is, I still don't even know what Depakote was supposed to treat.

I have been down this road so many times before that I am tired of second-guessing doctors. I decided, long ago to simply follow their orders. I always hope that when a doctor says he has a drug that will heal me, it will.

Savella could be the miracle cure. Dr. Olivera might have the key to ridding me of all this pain. He is a neurologist, which means he is super smart. He could be the key.

But the events following the initial prescription are some of the worst and most erratic times. It is similar to the Lexapro days of my first August in Los Angeles but much worse. (See Appendix T.)

The Poet

He is a fellow creative writing major, I should have known. Brent walks in late to the roundtable discussion. There are only a handful of us, Jakob to my right and Jakob's sorority sister to my left. (Oops, sorry Jakob). It is his super bitchy in-a-sorority friend. I see a tall, dark-haired boy in black, ripped jeans carrying a Rock-star energy drink enter the class. He obnoxiously pulls a chair out of the stack in the corner, realizes everyone is staring at him and interrupts the professor.

"Hey!" he shouts. I lose all focus as I fall into the idea of this very interesting character.

The professor sharply asks him to take a seat, "Good of you to be on time."

"Yeah of course! I couldn't wait for class-time!" He's smiling wide, making me burst out laughing, along with...wait, no one else.

Well I think he's funny.

I shrink into my seat a little bit. He glances at me.

"She's thinks I'm funny," the guy says.

"Okay, let's get back to the Victorian poets. Can som—" the professor starts.

Fuck the Victorians, they're super annoying. The Romantics are so much more relatable.

"Fuck. I hate those assholes," the boy says as if he has Tourette's.

The professor uncrosses his arms and smacks them down onto the table.

"Can we all refrain from commenting, please."

"Yup, I'm assuming you're talking to me. And yes, of course, sir," the new guy says.

Okay, I've got to get to know this guy.

I kick Jakob under the table. He always knows everyone…everywhere. He brushes me off like a fly buzzing around a horsetail.

"Jakob!" I jab him in the side with my pointy elbow. "Who is that?" I whisper.

"Kali, do you have anything to offer our discussion today?" the professor asks.

Well of course I do. I love being put on the spot like this. It's like a challenge.

"Sure!" I say.

"Great. Enlighten us," the professor says and motions with his hand to proceed.

"Well, I agree that the Victorians suck. However, Rossetti is really interesting to me, almost timeless. She is able to convert honest emotion, subtly, yet aggressively…" I ramble on into a somewhat coherent argument.

After someone vehemently disagrees with my point, I get to sit back and relax. My talking for the day is done. I scribble a couple words onto a piece of notebook paper and draw a huge arrow toward the rock-star boy. "Who is that?"

"I don't know! I'll ask Camille after," Jakob angry whispers to me. Jakob is annoyed for one reason or another. He'd been acting super snooty lately.

"Brent," the guy next to Camille whispers, "he's cool."

I guess he saw my sign!

Jasper in Los Flores

I liked that Brent would come over in the middle of the night and make jewelry with me. Sitting on the floor of my craziest apartment yet, he told me that he loved the layout.

In an Adderall-fueled haze we would craft necklaces and discuss poetry, along with ideas about foreign films we loved, our ideas on *La Règle du Jeu*, my favorite film.

The first night he came over, he rode his white Vespa all the way from Los Flores, bearing gifts: a pair of mini rifle charms that he'd taken from his friend Jasper.

Jasper was the most lavish character of a person. I thought his accent was also real, but it wasn't. He drove a huge BMW sedan, brand new, owned this old nightclub, and had to be at least thirty, though it turns out he was younger than me.

Jasper's mother would buy a rotisserie chicken every night and have Jasper handfeed it to her tea-cup poodle. I know this because I was given the task one night and was scolded by Jasper when the chicken got cold because I left the door to the mansion's master bedroom's balcony open. I had been sitting outside sipping the drink he had made me, gazing into the brilliance of all the lights below. We must have been at the very top of the hill.

Jasper doesn't drink. But one night, he took us to an underground Vietnamese place. He swore it would be the best time of our lives; transcendental, I think he had said.

Upon entering, I realize that everyone is glowing in the black-light. An enormous number of people are actually dancing under a disco-ball. The empty tables in the restaurant are, I guess, where they serve Thai food by day.

It isn't two minutes after I enter the place that a nicely dressed business man grabs my hand, interlaces my fingers with his, squeezes my hand and leads me to a bathroom. Outside, a huge, black man, a bodyguard, stands, arms- crossed, looking like he means business.

The door opens and a pair falls out laughing.

A man shouts from inside, "Come!"

I don't have time to think before he's laying out a line of coke on the back of his hand.

Wow, this is a really nice bathroom.

"It's on me. You're too beautiful to pay," the man says.

The nicely dressed man in the bathroom carefully lays out a new line of cocaine. He looks like he could be a friend of my father's, completely non-threatening. After offering me about five more lines, he looks at me with a certain glimmer of something in his eyes.

"Sweetheart." He pauses, his pupils slightly dancing from the left to right as he studies me, "Go have some fun now."

He pushes open the door, grabs my hand and leads me out of the door. I'm like a limp child being dragged around the mall.

Brent is beaming when he sees me. "You went in the back, right?" Brent asks.

"What the heck? This place is amazing!" I say.

"They put it in the Thai iced tea too," he says.

"Wait, how? ... Or, why?!" I say.

Brent speaks louder now in order to be heard over the music, "And they're open until six a.m.," Brent says. He grabs my hand and hastily leads me into the surge of people on the dance floor.

We end up at Jasper's house, five in the morning. Jasper is filming me with an old-fashioned camera. Mascara's dripping down my face. Brent and I are laughing hysterically about nothing in Jasper's steam-room shower.

DR. FIASCHETTI: JULY 20, 2011
Nuvigil. (See Appendix U.)

Brent Is on Drugs, Or He Was...

"What!" Brent yells and hits the binder I am carrying out of my hands. It comes crashing down onto the wood floor, making him laugh even louder at the dramatic scene he's causing. "Fuck your binder!" he yells proceeding to destroy my carefully organized rolling clothes rack. He rips my RucKus dress off the rack. He picks his high tops up off the ground, throwing them at the canvas Christina painted for me.

"Let's get fucking wasted, bro!" Brent yells and kicks the rack to the ground. It slams into Stella's cage, forcing Stella to slink out.

"What are you doing? Stop!" I yell.

"Whatever the fuck I want!" Brent makes sure his voice is louder than mine. He bends over, shoveling through the mess of clothing. "Where the fuck is my jacket? My favorite fucking jacket."

"I don't know," I say.

"I need a fucking cigarette, and they're in my jacket. Where the fuck is my coat?" Brent isn't angry, but rather, crazed.

"Brent, please stop. You can have one of mine," I say.

He jumps up so quickly that I stumble backward. He grabs my shoulders. "Relax, baby girl. I've got you."

His eyes lock with mine. He jolts me backward and then yanks me back forward so that I'm upright again. I struggle to maintain my footing. He jolts me backward once more. "See? I'm just kidding!"

The thing that was previously stabilizing Brent just enough to make me think his "crazy" is like mine is either not working, or working triple time. All I know is that my crazy isn't nuts. It is self-aware: an act, almost. Moreso, a willingness to embrace my full self, the artist within, no barriers.

After many questions, I finally get Brent to admit that he has been given a new pill: Savella. Yup. Savella. The same drug that drove me out of my mind, for real crazy: the kind of crazy where I got into a car with a complete stranger at Rite Aid, leaving my brand new Beach Cruiser unlocked on the street because I was tired.

It was fun to throw Red Stripe bottles off of my balcony, yeah, but this wasn't fun anymore.

It is fun discussing the universe and beading ridiculous necklaces at three a.m., pretending to audition for reality shows, at one point, needing a name for our team and on camera, deciding to call our team the Black Widows.

I feed off of his vibrantly-ridiculous "no fucks given" energy. But it isn't fun to watch him march into my neighbor's home with his fists clenched in a rage, knowing that Brent will get the shit beat out of him if he tries to touch this guy.

Yeah, Vegas for his grandparents' anniversary is fun, but finding him posted up in the bathtub when I finally get a ride down to Newport, that is odd. Brent grew up in a different part of Orange County, but rented a villa in Newport Coast on occasion. The beachside villa was down the street from my childhood home.

There is literally a house full of wild college kids drinking excessively expensive alcohol in a suite at Pelican Hill and I can't find Brent anywhere. An asshole is trying to corner me in a bedroom. I duck underneath him, and bust into the bathroom by accident to find Brent drinking a glass of whiskey, listening to his favorite Morrissey album. He is sporting a freshly dead skunk hairstyle: white on the sides, shaved close, and black and poofy long up top (his mother was a hair stylist).

"Well hello there, Kali, are you enjoying the party?" Brent asks.

I kind of dug the way he pretended to be an English rock star, but also kind of worried he thought he was an English rock star.

Sitting on the cobbled steps outside my studio apartment, I ask Brent what he wants to do with his life. The point is to figure out where he is coming from lately, in all of his newfound insanity.

For me, the craziness is surface-level. I've always understood my deeper purpose. This is the one vein that runs through my entire life. No matter how crazy my mind is, or how insane I act on impulse, I know what I am here on this planet to do.

Brent's answer signs, seals and delivers itself, directly into my lap. "I want to be the most fucked up guy at the party."

A cigarette hangs out the side of his mouth. The nicotine patch begins to burn my arm and make me feel sick.

"I am being serious," I say, unamused.

"Seriously, I'd like to be just so fucked up all the time, be the most fucked-up dude and like never get sober," Brent says.

He hasn't always been like this.

"You know, Savella drove me out of my mind," I say.

"I fucking love it!" he says. His eyes widen with the statement. "I took double today, and I'm going to take more when I get back inside."

"Please don't take that stuff," I say.

His laugh is piercing…

Before this, I enjoyed that Brent's "crazy" outdid my "crazy." Nothing is too off-the-wall for him, nothing. But the longer I spend around him, the more I realize that his crazy is very much for real. It isn't a game for him. And now, he is scaring me. It is only after Brent describes his fantasy that I finally heed my poetry professor's warning to steer clear of him.

"I'd love to fuck you while I shove your face into the fan and watch the blood splatter onto the walls like a painting," Brent says.

I think he is kidding.

He has to be…duh! You're so funny Brent.

I stare into his eyes, seeking to find what he is saying. It can't possibly be real. But I don't get the answer I want. His eyes are vacant. Brent looks far different from the guy I met outside English class, asking me if he could hear some of my poetry and proceeding to accompany me to my poetry reading. I think back to meeting Brent:

"There's no way I'm letting you read to all those poetry assholes without me," Brent said. He even held my books as we navigated through the commanding brick buildings under the bright California sun that turned the grass into a sort of fairy-tale backdrop.

Today, I look into Brent's eyes, in my second-story, no air-conditioning, sectioned into different kinds of studios, apartment, and he looks scary. The black eyeliner he wears under his eyes is thicker than usual.

Why is he laughing like that?

DR. FIASCHETTI: AUGUST 17, 2011
Rx Antabuse (See Appendix V.)

Brent Is Nuts, For Real

Brent decides to bring all of his things from his parents' house, where he's been staying after taking a quarter off to "get his head together" and throw them into my tiny studio apartment. After piling them on my desk, he starts neatly hanging each piece on my desk chair, announcing: "I'll stay here!"

He waves to his father from my second-level apartment on Carmelina.

"Okay, it's a bit small for all of that," I say.

"You said I could stay," Brent says.

"Yeah, for a couple of nights…without luggage. I don't even have a closet here," I say.

I live in a new place on the same street. It is much smaller than my first apartment down the street, and a lot hotter. A savvy saleswoman offered to drive me to the available apartments, gushing about the wood floors and the view and seducing me into renting this terrible apartment up the street from my last place.

The reality of how small the apartment is does not hit me until I try to bring in my bathroom and kitchen. There is a two-by-four-foot offset into a two-by-two room with a toilet and janky, mini shower. The grout is crumbling. It is bad. In a nut moment, I forgot to even ask about air conditioning. So here I am, in a mini oven of an apartment.

Inspired by the novelty of it all, I decide to make my studio apartment live up to its name and divide it into all of the things I want to accomplish here: four sections. I make it an actual art studio.

I section off my music side, with my keyboard, guitar, and notebooks, then my fashion area, with a rolling rack of clothing and scraps and beads torn off random vintage finds, and then there is the painting (mostly for Christina) section, and my bed, which can be pushed against the wall vertically during the day to allow for more room in my dancing part of the studio.

I am in love with it. And then, my parents arrive. My mother is not happy. She is furious. Around the third day, when I realize just how hot the apartment becomes without air conditioning, I know my mother is right. I need to get the fuck out. And, right as I make that decision, Brent sets up shop.

> Fuck my life.
> I thought I was done with him.
> "What? You don't like me anymore?" Brent says, tilting his head back and forth like an annoying bird on something. His eyes look crazy. He mocks my concern, mimicking me. "Oh my God." He laughs loudly. "Stop doing drugs. You are acting insane."
> "Whatever, Brent," I say.
> Good thing I'm moving in three days…
> He's not getting a key.

Under the Lights:...Camera, Action!

"Are you busy tonight?"

I laugh and take a sip of my Jack and Coke. "Who are you?"

This guy, wearing a very cute sweater and dress shirt poking up out of the neckline, pulls a notepad out of his back pocket and begins to write. He leans on the side of the rooftop bar for a writing surface. Good move. The drunk, college kids who have been lining up all night to karaoke have just been given the first go ahead of the night. There is been no way I could heard him. And I am way too tired from the week prior to try and make a "lean in and put my mouth basically on your ear to hear me" moment.

Off-key harmonies ring loudly through the dark red bar. The pool tables are already covered in abandoned drinks and the crowd is rowdy.

I look back over at Brent and his friend from out of town, who is surprisingly normal. Brent, however, is not. He is currently in crazy mode, acting obnoxiously as usual. I watch as he repeatedly pushes his way too thin frame off the nearest pool table, laughing hysterically, head flung back, teeth gritting, as he attempts to hoist himself above the crowd for no apparent reason. It is karaoke for God's sake.

I feel this nicely dressed guy grab my arm and I look back at him. The note reads:

"I'm Julian. We are filming a movie next door. Are you available?"

Before I have a chance to think twice, I'm basically grabbing Julian by the arm, headed out. "Yes! I'm down." I suck in as much alcohol as possible in this next anxiety-filled gulp.

"Great," Julian says, grabbing for my drink. I pull it back into me. "We have plenty next door."

I clutch it tighter.

"I promise," he says confidently.

His Bambi-eyes and Gucci cologne melt away any doubt as I turn into putty in his assumingly lotioned hands. This guy must be Puerto Rican. He's beautiful.

And strong!

The tug of his hand yanks me through the densest part of the crowd. His fingers tighten around mine and I relax into his grip. I can only see his silver watch and feel the cashmere of his sweater as I am swooped through the mess into the cool night air.

I laugh as the moon lights up the night. In a moment, joy washes over me. I love this guy. The loud bar contrasts brilliantly with the stifled silence of the night.

"Follow me," Julian says. He's holding out his hand again, almost confused by my letting go.

Swoon…I giggle in awe of his cuteness. His smile is perfect too.

"Wait! The Brendon! How did you—" I start.

Okay, so this is a legit film.

I sober up as the light coming from the main camera blasts in my direction.

"Cut! Makeup please!" the director shouts.

I sweat a little more as the several makeup artists throw on booties and carefully step onto the set: each one going to their respective actors.

I'm chosen first. She smiles as she applies concealer enthusiastically, with the largest concealer brush I'd ever seen. Next, she swoops under my eyes, finishing with a new swipe of lip gloss.

"Am I good?" I ask hesitantly, staring into her eyes as if they're mirrors. We don't have a mirror close to set and I can't get off the meticulously placed barstool to run to the makeshift dressing-room.

"You look beautiful," she says reassuringly.

For a moment I think we are friends rather than acquaintances.

"Kali!" the director, Spenser, shouts from his seat behind the camera moving on the track. "Can you read for Ms. Greenwood?"

"Yes!" I say.

"Light her please!" the director shouts.

All the sudden, I am the star of the film. I squint as the lights move closer. Good thing I only had a couple drinks before being ripped away. I'll sweat them both out by the top of the hour.

My love-interest is model-quality, stage make-up and all. His blue eyes are unreal with his swooping blonde locks. "I'm Brian," he says.

"Hi, Brian, Kali," I say and hold out my hand awkwardly, a reflex that I'm really wishing I hadn't formed. He grabs my hand like a gentlemen, correcting everything.

"Very nice to meet you, Kali. I'm glad you stumbled in here," Brian says.

"Spenser! Why are you trying her?!" the brunette lead is shouting at the director. "Does she even act, Spenser?! Where did you find her?! The bar?!" Spencer doesn't reply. "This is bullshit," the brunette says. She stomps toward the dressing-room collecting her stuff, "Fucking amateurs!"

She is unrealistically perfect-looking. Her movie-star waves put my natural highlights and beachy-straight hair to shame. I look like a kid in comparison.

I am just getting comfortable with the new stage direction when I hear a familiar voice that fills me with dread. I squint to look out past the lights to see him.

"Kali!" Brent shouts like a madman. Security is holding him back at the door.

"Come get me. They won't let me past," he says, crazed. I look toward Spencer and he catches my despair.

"Excuse me, this is a closed set. Everyone not working on the film needs to leave now or the authorities will be involved," Spencer says.

Spencer motions toward his personal security and then readjusts himself, looking back into the telescope lens of the camera.

"Kali, you ready?" Spencer asks.

I squint in an attempt to block out the blinding lights of the set. I smile, excited to impress my new friends;

"Born ready."

Species: September 3, 2011:

Well Brent said it would be funny,
to watch the blood
from my battered face
spray the ceiling.
For some reason,
I thought he had to be kidding.
But when the choking started,
life got a little more deceiving.
I don't think that I am of the same species.

Am I running
Am I running again?
Racing through terminals,
keeping my eyes on the ground.
I glance at you,
you smile.
But what I really need,
is another dose of denial.
Blame it on the mother,
Blame it on the father,
Blame it on the brother,
or the older sister.
Why couldn't you have…
Why couldn't they have…
Why couldn't he live with the fact that I may just
be a little bit wild.

3. Epilogue Not Only Are My Doctors Famous (*Losing Kali Joke*), So Are My Attackers

Aaron's Article

A few years after I'd forgotten about Aaron, something interesting happened. I was taking the trash out at the barre gym (I worked at one day a week for free SoulCycle classes) when the face I once knew so well started moving toward me like an illusion. I thought I was hallucinated him.

I was thankful that it was still light outside as he passed by me so closely I could feel the movement of air hit my body like a cement wall. I shuddered the moment I passed him and registered that he was, in fact, a real human form. I did a double-take, catching my breath, as if I hadn't breathed since the day I woke up on that windowsill.

The classic khaki, "asshole" shorts, Sperrys and navy Lacoste shirt, paired with the arrogant way his hands were shoved into his pockets, gave me the answer: Yes. It was him.

I nearly ran back to the gym. I was the last person there for the night. I quickly locked the door, and felt a surge of terror.

In a moment of pure instinct, I typed his name into the web browser. Several articles popped up plastered with his obnoxious face: dumb pictures with drunk girls. I click further, not believing the gruesome headline. It expands into an article depicting, basically, a monster.

Aaron was not a first-time offender. A simple Google search of his name pulled up a strain of articles all depicting awful beatings of women.

He had been arrested several times for these gruesome attacks, raping and beating girlfriends. The articles not only depicted these events as traumatic but terrifying.

One article described the police showing up at his Beverly Hills home after he strangled and threatened to kill his girlfriend a few months before.

"Charged with attempted murder ... 'I'm going to kill you tonight'... brutally beating ... battered and bloody..." Phrases describing the attacks fall off the screen like tears, as I forget to breathe. I am overwhelmed by the sheer amount and scope of his aggression toward women. He just keeps doing it, victim after victim.

No one stopped this guy. I didn't stop this guy.

Event after event, six in total, official Los Angeles Police Department records. Each of those incidents occurred with a different girlfriend and were severe enough to have police either come to his Beverly Hills home or arrest him on the spot.

How many other women did he hurt?

My "Welcome to the City" night with Aaron took place years before these police reports.

The crimes had simply gotten more and more gruesome over time. And I felt my insides turn to ice and then the blood in my veins surged through me from every angle.

I COULD HAVE FOLLOWED THROUGH AT THE POLICE STATION THAT DAY. But I had been afraid that maybe it had been my fault, or maybe my crazy mind had just imagined the entire thing, or maybe I didn't remember anything because I'd subconsciously blocked it out.

But the truth has always been the same; I knew what had happened to me, and I knew now that these kinds of people never stop with just one. They never do.

I chose, for my own sanity, to think that this time was special, specific to me.

I chose to believe that I was the only person this guy would have done this to and he had done it for a specific reason, to get back at me for not paying him enough attention. Or maybe because I was annoying and young and stupid and I parked the wrong way in the insanely steep driveway of his Beverly Hills home. Or maybe it was because I had spilled on his rug that one time, or because I simply had gotten the wrong idea, and this is how things really worked in life. That women were actually treated liked this normally, that I was not an exception, but just oversensitive.

Then I'd get a flashback to waking up that morning in so much pain, bleeding, and knowing he had raped me the night prior. Stumbling around his room, when he wouldn't even wake up or move the huge, poofy, comforter, luxuriously wrapped around his boyish body.

He looked so innocent there.

Within months, I reacted by deciding it was my fault, feeling bad for him, since he was from back East and said he had nowhere to go for Thanksgiving, and I actually invited him to our family Thanksgiving, where, no joke, my mother felt bad for the guy and urged me to take him to our local beach before heading back to the city.

I wanted to scream to the entire house how much I hated this man, that I had no idea why I had invited him here and the fact that my sister had let him borrow her University of Indiana sweatshirt made me want to throw up all over this guy's blonde curls.

I hated his Topsiders that used to be my favorite style of shoe in high school. And I hated his baby pink Lacoste shirt, idiotically rolled up at the sleeves for no reason except to showcase his awkwardly short biceps that were toned, but just fucking awkwardly small.

I hated his stupid khaki shorts and that dumb metal ring belt that made him look like such an East Coast heartthrob when really he was just an awkward asshole who my dad hated from the moment they met.

Aaron had sold me my first apartment. He wore Whitestrips on his teeth while touring the building with us. He got my information and Facebooked me before I had even left the city.

"Why would a guy wear Whitestrips while showing an apartment? Like, dude, talk them off beforehand. Weird guy, Kali," my dad said in the car on the way home. "Huh, Kali," my dad repeated for emphasis, wondering why his daughter seemed to be in a trance staring out the passenger-seat window.

"Oh…yeah, for sure…" I said. "That guy was weird for sure."

I was distracted by the messages in my messenger account from Aaron, this actor/real estate agent/older, more mature than Jaxx-guy.

Jason's Article

After finding articles about Dr. Morano§§, Cathy*** , and Aaron, I hold my breath, and search the internet for the few other people who came into my life at a time when I was especially vulnerable, and were especially devious. One in particular.

I remember him mentioning that he had changed his name, but it hit! He lives in New York City.

Sure enough, Jason checks out to be a complete asshole. I find a single article he wrote where he explains, as a personal trainer, how he gets clients to sign expensive contracts with him.

He goes into detail, dissecting the ways he is able to discover each person's real reason for working out. Jason explains how he aims to find the client's deepest insecurities and then use those deep-seated insecurities to keep them coming back, reminding them of their inadequacies and mock-supporting them through said insecurities all the while.

He's obviously oblivious to the immorality of it all.

Each of women he writes about, he says, essentially came to see him to have sex with him. And Jason describes the ways he manipulates simple stretches to put himself into a sort-of mounting position.

---

§§ This doctor had had his license suspended twice and was hospitalized at one point for medicating himself with his own medication samples. See *Losing Kali*, Book 1 in the Finding Kali trilogy.

*** A doctor in *Losing Kali* who I saw to with Jaxx. She prescribed a boatload three, extremely dangerous medications in huge quantities. She is now in prison facing thirty years to life for murder.

He practices displaying masculine dominance over his clients by intensifying, for no physical benefit to the client, their physical interactions to mock sex poses. He describes each client, and her character-specific ways of trying to seduce him. He writes about a few stereotypes: the lonely trophy-wife, slutty sorority girl, stuck in the closet (specifically because he is a cop) gay guy, and lastly, the girl who went to my school who now has a very successful position in the music industry. He says she blurts out: "When can we stretch again?" after every single session with him.

In each case, he describes women who just want to fuck him.

Afterword

My dad recently said to me, "You were a very self-aware crazy person. It was interesting. You knew how crazy you were acting. You'd say: 'I know I'm being crazy right now, but…' So you knew." And this is the crucial difference between someone who can barely make it out alive and someone who has been given just a bit too much and can't see the problem anymore.

It is frightening that so many people in our country are playing the edge on this, with multiple drugs at the same time.

Side Effects Include Death

Today, this beautiful Thursday morning, I have the day off, it's eight a.m. and I'm still in bed. A very familiar commercial comes on. A woman, in her kitchen, blue-eyes, worry lines between them, speaks about an ailment that has held her back. It was B.E.D. Binge eating disorder. I see the graphic of a pizza pop up on the screen, and I already know there will be a pharmaceutical company claiming to cure this chemical imbalance.

This familiar lady clears things up by saying that her disorder used to claim her life and now she's taken back power by adhering to her doctor's orders of taking medicine to cure the chemical imbalance that triggers her lack of control.

A few moments later, I see a female ex-athlete, sitting on the red leather couch next to the main female news anchor of the most popular morning show in the country. She asks potent questions, but this woman simply doesn't answer them; she just reverts back to her state of unrest and distress. She claims pretzels were a trigger food, and when asked about the similarity to bulimia, she talks about the sadness she experienced while trying on bridesmaids dresses.

A photograph slowly expands to fit the screen. She looks about forty pounds heavier in the picture than she does now. The photograph of her in her pale bridesmaid tube dress is supposed to represent the pain she experienced due to her B.E.D. and the fluctuating weight that ensued.

This interview's so coached and neatly folded that it could fit into every woman's knock-off Boho wallet across the nation. She wears a pale blue sweater over grayish slacks. She is the epitome of classy but understated. I see through the bullshit immediately and hate her for playing the part.

I wonder how much money Pfizer paid her to be there. How many times they rehearsed how to answer such invasive questions. Surely no one would ever answer the bulimia question on the No. 1 rated morning news show.

It's an unwritten rule that people on Channel 7 in the morning don't talk about real emotions or circumstances. If they are going to try, they are quaint and quiet with their statements.

Good Morning America simply cannot allow unvarnished realness to impinge on their belly laughter and cozy comments to one another as they pass it "on over to you, Al. How are the fans out there?"

Let me tell you a little bit about the drug they are marketing to middle-aged women across the country. Vyvanse was the first stimulant I ever took. It was prescribed to Jaxx for ADD. Who knows what the real issue was; it was not like he worked any harder in school or could concentrate better when he took it. He just had it.

I ended up using Vyvanse because as a stimulant, it cuts off your appetite. And name one woman who is against losing her appetite completely for most of the day, and regaining it just like normal for dinner. It's a miracle.

When I went to my psychiatrist and told her how well Vyvanse worked—my ability to concentrate got stronger and my impulse control got better—she explained that she disliked Vyvanse. She said that would not be her first option, that it was made for children, but had been recalled. She felt strongly that there was a less intense option. And this doctor wasn't exactly conservative in her approach.

You see, the thing that bothers me most about these kinds of blatant ploys for dependence is that they aren't just pandering to the doctors now and dictating what the doctors should be giving their patients; they are now also pleading with the public in order to produce new patients, who might never have stepped into their doctor's office without having seen this charming, seemingly victorious woman on *Good Morning America*, who had been through so much but had finally found the one pill that solved her problem.

This is just purely unfair and manipulative. The way in which every answer to each question was riddled with emotion is just criminal.

"When in doubt, talk about your feelings," the big pharma execs probably coached.

"Just think back to when you weighed one sixty. How did you feel about yourself? Were you happy that you had just eaten a pint of Haagen Dazs?"

That's the common thread with these commercials. When the medicine is for men, they play on sexy women, fancy cars, and elbow grease. The backdrop of a gray-haired, forty-year-old, fixing his own car and then driving it down a desert road, showing off not only his manly ability to be self-sufficient but also his "unchained" lifestyle; no one and no thing is holding him back.

Did you pick up on the idea that taking this pill would actually make you less self-sufficient? I'll bet you didn't even think of it. That's due to the genius of advertising. They show you the exact opposite of what is actually happening in reality. Then they advertise a pill at the end that should allow for the fantasy to become your reality. You know it's stupid, yet the images stick. I mean, that guy was so ripped though.

For women, our battle is different. For us, the appeal is to empathy and our lack of ability to properly attend to our families when we are not in the right mindset.

Light pierces through the dark bedroom. She's still in bed. She sits up, shoulders hunched, sad-faced. A golden retriever enters, dropping his tennis ball in front of the gray-faced, messy-haired woman. She just looks away. The dog slowly walks out, sans tennis ball.

Later, the medicine is discovered! She's out on a walk! Her hair is washed and she's even throwing the tennis ball down the road. She bends down and vivaciously rubs the beautifully groomed golden as she laughs, probably at how embarrassing she was acting earlier!

Or they project a lonesome woman cartoon, looking glum, walking into a conference room with her head down. Oh man, she's so weak!

And later, they mention the medicine. The music changes and she's at home, a beautiful cartoon home. She walks, head held high, right out through the sliding glass doors into the grass-filled backyard over to her handsome husband who is manning the grill. He grins lovingly at her as she sets the plate of condiments down for her three energetic teenage boys. She's a new woman! She works all day, we'll surmise in a better state than before, and comes home to make dinner, happily for her clichéd American family. In this the kind of family, when the boys talk back to her, she laughs.

"Well that isn't very nice is it, Dillon," she says. She's the perfectly meek woman *and* she contributes in the workplace.

The Facts about Pharmaceuticals, Educate Yourself

This is a time when awareness is growing that the ability to heal ourselves comes from within. With this realization should come great joy and a sense of self-sufficiency, even power. Wellness offices are popping up all across the country.

When this advancement occurs, the men profiting from our dependence on prescription medications suffer. They find that their stock values are dropping and they need to quickly find a way to turn a higher profit.

So these brilliant men—instead of going into wellness or more holistic approaches to health, —decide to lie. They decide to remove warnings about side-effects or negative reactions, rename the drug, and release a new advertising campaign along. This campaign includes barrage of sponsored conferences where physicians are paid to speak on behalf of said drug after a twenty-one-year-old pharmaceutical rep gave them samples of the drug and essentially bribed them to prescribe and endorse it.

Instead of moving forward with positive change, executives have dug their heels in, demanding that nothing change, especially their income. So they get creative and flipped the system on its head. They began developing a disease or imbalance to fit an old recipe. They began clumping common symptoms together and naming them, offering up their drug as a solution and pushing it into the briefcases of the medical professionals and the purses of the affluent.

This happened with fibromyalgia, as I'm writing this I can hear the commercial saying, "generalized, widespread pain" that doesn't get better with sitting or standing." What the heck! If you are in pain, everywhere, all the time, and it is common enough for there to be a commercial about a drug for it, we have far too many people still in the workplace.

I got shingles in fifth grade, well, more like three shingles.

They are a result of a compromised immune system. You think that possibly there are more cases of shingles due to the things, including medicine and food, we put into our bodies??

Like many other drug commercials, the ad for the shingles vaccine is produced to resemble a public service announcement. It presents a condition and shows people telling how awful the sickness is and how badly it hurts. Even the strongest men, such as a retired firefighter, suffer horribly from this condition. Then the pharmaceutical company's logo comes on the screen, and a serious, authoritative tells you to ask your doctor about your risk of getting the virus.

The company is presenting a problem that will need treatment when it strikes. You are told that when this bad omen comes about, it will tear you apart, and the first thing you must do is go to the doctor and ask about AstraZeneca. Maybe they can give you some opioid pain-killers while you're there, or possibly diagnose you with anxiety, if you are worried about your illness.

Or maybe, if you can't sleep at night due to the burning of the shingles virus, you actually have an underlying condition, such as restless leg syndrome that would need to be treated with a prescription for Ambien. Ambien is the butterfly medication or is that Lyrica?

Hmmm, anyway, you're gonna get shingles, and then you'll need to ask your doctor about AstraZeneca to make sure it goes away. That is the deal. Basically you need to donate to their foundation. It's a perfect plan because you donate directly through taking unneeded medications that they dramatically sell to you by playing your emotions like a digital keyboard.

Confused?

Me too.

Manipulating the Patients

There are enough people feeling out of sorts and reaching for mood-stabilizers, anxiety medications, antidepressants, and painkillers for our nation to be seriously and consistently working on a solution. Why, when I was taking antibiotics regularly, was I ending up in the hospital six times a year with severe kidney problems? (Topamax). How come for the months after using an alternative form of treatment I haven't visited the ER once? Not one time.

Part of this falls on the shoulders of the patients. When you have an expectation that you need a certain substance in order to recover, there is pressure on the doctor to prescribe that substance or risk losing you as a patient. Obviously, the stand-up doctor should always only prescribe something he feels is completely and utterly needed to heal, but more often that not, I've been in a room where a doctor simply cannot identify the problem and so he treats the entire body with a round of antibiotics to just about kill everything living inside of you.

I've also been on that couch when the doctor simply says: "What do you think the best route to take is?"

I answer with my choice prescriptions, and the doctor fills them. No questions asked. I've also been through the fifteen-minute appointment system, where the doctor goes through a checklist of questions like: "Do you feel the impulse to hurt others or yourself?"

In which case, you answer however you feel you need to, in order to move along to the next question and get the prescription you want.

This is a broken system, fueled by the monetary gain of the pharmaceutical companies who can jack up their prices once they are confident a prescription has the perfect balance of addictive qualities and super-charged chemical compounds. Meaning, you feel better due to a surge in one chemical all at once, and then cannot physically re-create the same surge without that exact same drug present in your system.

Worse than that, once the medicine is taken away, you not only are dragged through hell in order to readjust your body to function properly without the chemical. As a result, the body goes into shutdown mode, not knowing how the heck to respond to such a change, and you go through everything from gaining five pounds a day even while working out twice a day intensely and eating far under a thousand calories.

There is also a mental side to equation. You begin to hate your body. You feel consistently tired. You aren't sick, but you'd rather be sick, so you can lie in bed all day because you have no motivation, no reason to get out of bed.

The people who put you into grip you are held in should be legally prosecuted to the fullest extent of the law. They are ruining lives prescribing by toxic chemicals to otherwise healthy human beings. In the process they condemn patients to either 1) suffer through ten years of hell in order to get back to where they started (suffering the original symptoms they sought help for in the first place) or 2) give up and start taking the medication again, swearing not to increase the dosage and promising not to take it for more than a couple months, though all the odds stacked against them.

I lost everything in an attempt to find solid ground.

APPENDICES

APPENDIX A

RX FX APPENDIX: LEXAPRO (ESCITALOPRAM)

If Kanye West refers to the withdrawal from this drug on an album, then you know it is for real.

> A variety of antidepressants have been reported to induce mania, including selective serotonin reuptake inhibitors, tricyclic antidepressants, monoamine oxidase inhibitors, venlafaxine, and nefazodone. In addition, mania induction has also been reported upon the withdrawal of antidepressant (FDA 2017).

I am prescribed Lexapro the same month I move to Los Angeles. It is the same month I leave home for the first time to make a life for myself in "The Hills." It is my time to fly.

Lexapro pretty much ruins this for me. The excessive drinking doesn't help. The two together, are, well, almost a successful suicide. My blackouts are frequent and while I am blacked-out, things are dangerous for me, to say the least.

I find dozens of articles about people taking Lexapro and drinking that explain my frequent blackouts and alcohol cravings. There is even an alternative medicine center offering to help when people off Lexapro. Its website lists the following symptoms:

> "anxiety, aggression, brain zaps, blurred vision, crying spells, cramps, concentration impairment, constipation, dizziness, diarrhea, depersonalization, electric shock like sensations, flu-like symptoms, flatulence, fatigue, gait instability, hostility, hallucinations, indigestion, insomnia, irritability, impaired speech, jumpy nerves, lethargy, lack of coordination, migraines, headaches, nervousness, nausea, paranoia, repetitive thoughts, pacing, sensory disturbances, severe internal restlessness (akathasia), tremors, tingling sensations, tinnitus, visual hallucinations, illusions, delusions, vivid dreams, troubling thoughts, worsened depression and speech/visual changes" (Alternative 2017).

Looking back on this traumatic period of my life, I recognize these symptoms from the horrifying few months at my first apartment. The things that happened, but also the things I did (swallowed a bottle of Xanax while dressed like Twiggy, which actually just consisted of drawing eyelashes on my face with an eyeliner pencil and wearing boots).

I always blamed my own mind for these treacherous times. I thought most of the things were in reaction to the trauma I had experienced. Maybe some were; however, reading these articles and comments from fellow victims makes me realize how much of a bonfire we are truly playing around when we mess with the chemicals in our brains.

The month I was prescribed Lexapro, I:

- Got drunk with a group of probably twelve guys and girls and yelled "Fuck bathing suits!" as I got into an elevator completely naked.
- Got raped and beaten but don't remember a thing and invited my rapist to Thanksgiving dinner. (Said rapist is now in prison, convicted of rape and assault. I found this out by a simple search of his name on the internet years later).
- Got so depressed I seriously considered jumping off a second-floor balcony.
- Had moments I felt I was too broken to continue. For days I didn't get out of bed. These were the times that the real me came back into the Lexapro-possessed me, and felt the weight of what had gone down in the past weeks.

This is the black box warning that The Food and Drug Administration [FDA] forced Lexapro to display on its medication guide and packaging:

> WARNINGS: The development of a potentially life-threatening serotonin syndrome or Neuroleptic Malignant Syndrome (NMS)-like reactions have been reported with SNRIs and SSRIs alone, including Celexa treatment, but particularly with concomitant use of serotonergic drugs (including triptans) with drugs which impair metabolism of serotonin (including MAOIs), or with antipsychotics or other dopamine antagonists… (FDA 2009).

Not to mention, the manufacturers of Lexapro, Forest Laboratories, also manufactur Celexa and Levothroid (a medication for Hashimotos, hypothyroidism). They were penalized in a combined $300 million penalty for distributing Levothroid before it was even approved by the FDA and also for marketing Celexa to children and adolescents when it was only approved for adults.

Celexa, Lexapro and Levothroid, all manufactured by Forest Laboratories, treat different conditions but were linked together in a $313-million penalty the manufacturer was forced to pay the U.S. government in 2010. Celexa is an antidepressant approved only for use in adults, but Forest promoted it as a safe drug for children and adolescents suffering from depression. The company distributed Levothroid when it was not yet approved by the FDA, and all three drugs were linked to false claims submitted to federal health care program (Drugwatch 2016).

APPENDIX B

RX FX: XANAX (ALPRAZOLAM)

I found the black box warning labeled "Use with Other CNS Depressants" particularly frightening:

> The benzodiazepines, including alprazolam (Xanax) produce additive CNS depressant effects when coadministered with other psychotropic medications, anticonvulsants, antihistaminics, ethanol and other drugs which themselves produce CNS depression (Drugs 2016).

APPENDIX C

RX FX VALIUM (DIAZEPAM)

In post-marketing experience, or the monitoring of the drug after it has been released into the marketplace there have been reports of:

> ...injury, Poisoning and Procedural Complications: There have been reports of falls and fractures in benzodiazepine users. The risk is increased in those taking concomitant sedatives (including alcoholic beverages) and in the elderly (FDA 2017).

APPENDIX D

RX FX: ATIVAN (LORAZEPAM)

Out of all the emotions I brought to the appointment with Dr. Thompson, the first therapist I ever saw, sadness is the one thing that I absolutely described to her that afternoon. Amazing, because the warnings/precautions label of the drug guide for Ativan says prescribing this drug may not only lead to dependency, but that it could make me more depressed.

> Preexisting depression may emerge or worsen; not for use with primary depressive disorder or psychosis … May impair mental/physical abilities. Use may lead to physical and psychological dependence … May have abuse potential … possible suicide in patients with depression; do not use in such patients without adequate antidepressant therapy (PDR 2016).

Dr. Thompson prescribes me Ativan after finding out that, on top of the real issue, I am a little bit afraid of elevators. In a case where my newly-diagnosed phobia [of elevators] does not disrupt anything in my life at all, why would someone prescribe this drug so easily? It is dangerous in adults, and has not even been properly tested for children. It seems that this doctor either had no idea she was playing with fire or did not care.

> Ativan should be used with extreme caution in CHILDREN younger than twelve years old; safety and effectiveness in these children have not been confirmed (Drugs 2016).

So, say Dr. Thompson was not thinking clearly when she prescribed me Ativan when I was eleven years old. Dr. Fiaschetti never did any sort of cognitive or intensive inquiry regarding my necessity for any sort of drug. But with the anti-anxiety medication alone, I had three to four different kinds at one time. She does not note this, of course, but my journal entries do and my mother, who kept one of the prescriptions with her, remembers this clearly.

Regardless of the necessity for an anxiety medication with serious side effects ESPECIALLY in an adolescent and ESPECIALLY in combination with the other medications, she prescribed them to me without ever reevaluating me for anything or even talking to me about how I felt. No one under the age of eighteen or actually, twenty-four, since that is the range found to have extreme increases in suicidality under the influence of these drugs, should ever be able to have three or four of these dangerous medications at one time. Especially if you are dealing with someone who is actually struggling with emotional or psychological issues. It's a recipe for disaster. And it was just that in my case.

Within days of my moving into my apartment in Los Angeles, my roommates called my mother after I, allegedly, I have no recollection of the first part, got drunk, took an entire bottle of Ativan, on top of the Seroquel, Lexapro I was taking. I decided that night, I remember this well, that I would dress up before going out. I would dress up as my favorite fashion icon, Twiggy I do remember carefully DRAWING on, no joke, DRAWing on my eyelashes, just like the famous photograph of Twiggy for Vogue, and stumbling in my high leg boots out of the bathroom. I don't remember the rest.

Ativan (lorazepam) is part of a group of drugs that are sometimes called skeletal muscle relaxants. They depress the central nervous system (Physicians Desk Reference [PDR] 2016). Ativan is also a sedative, an anti-anxiety medication belonging to the class of benzodiazepines (benzos), a class of drugs that would become all too familiar to me after this.

Ativan is a schedule IV drug. (Medshadow 2016) This category assignment says that Ativan's so-called risk of abuse is low, in comparison to say, Oxycontin, a Schedule II narcotic, or Vicodin, a little bit less addictive as a Schedule III narcotic. Adderall, for instance, is a Schedule II stimulant. Xanax and Valium are both in the same group of schedule IV benzos (Medshadow 2016). In doctor-speak, Ativan is relatively harmless. But that's far from the truth. In conjunction with other medicines or alcohol, Ativan can produce fatal results:

> Increased CNS-depressant effects with other CNS depressants (e.g., alcohol, barbiturates, antipsychotics, sedative/hypnotics, anxiolytics, antidepressants, narcotic analgesics, sedative antihistamines, anticonvulsants, anesthetics); may lead to potentially fatal respiratory depression (Physicians' Desk Reference [PDR] 2016).

APPENDIX E

RX FX: TOPAMAX (TOPIRAMATE)

- •AED THAT REQUIRES BLACK BOX ON SUICIDALITY

Topamax not only includes a boxed warning for suicidality, it also includes a boxed warning regarding a risk of serotonin syndrome and hypomania, not only upon administration, but upon discontinuation. We will stick to the kidney stones Topamax gave me in this book. See *Losing Kali*, Book 1 in the Finding Kali trilogy for experiences of the other two.

In a study to find if Topamax directly causes kidney stone formation, the conclusion is simple:

> Treatment with topiramate causes systemic metabolic acidosis, markedly lower urinary citrate excretion, and increased urinary pH. These changes increase the propensity to form calcium phosphate stones (Welch 2006).

Topamax is a member of the antiepileptic class of drugs that causes an increase in suicidality (FDA 2017).

To top it all off:

> The manufacturer, two subsidiaries of health care giant Johnson & Johnson, were found guilty of marketing the drug [Topamax] for unapproved treatments, such as weight loss and bipolar disorder. The Department of Justice fined Ortho-McNeil Pharmaceutical and Ortho- McNeil-Janssen Pharmaceuticals more than $81-million in 2010 for this dangerous practice (Drugwatch 2017).

APPENDIX F

RX FX SEROQUEL (QUETIAPINE FUMARATE)

- BLACK BOX WARNING FOR AND SUICIDALITY

Seroquel is an anti-psychotic drug that, in my circle alone, was taken by at least two people, including Jaxx's mother. Jaxx warned me about Seroquel because he'd watched his mother. He said it made her "fat."

I laughed it off until I remembered my mother's comment from the night prior regarding how much I'd been eating late at night.

"I've never seen you crave so much junk in my life!" she said as I shoved multiple slices of sourdough bread topped with chunks of melted cheddar cheese into my mouth.

I wiped away the oil from my mouth to ask the age-old question, "Do you think I'm fat, Mom?" under a late-night haze of Seroquel zombie-ness. I could barely make out her facial features because my eyesight stayed in a constant "just woke up" blur on Seroquel.

Guess what?

AstraZeneca paid $647-million to settle a global lawsuit alleging that Seroquel caused diabetes. "California will receive more than $5.2 million" (Wilson 2017).

How about that! It's even written in my medical charts that I craved sugar and carbohydrates late at night. It was prescribed to me to help with insomnia but looks like it's not even approved for this use. It is an anti-psychotic.

AstraZeneca paid another $68.5–million "as part of a multistate settlement over allegations that it promoted its psychiatric drug Seroquel for unapproved uses, such as treating insomnia and Alzheimer's disease" (Ceasar 2017).

> It is estimated that AstraZeneca will have paid a total of about $1.9-billion to defend against and settle the personal injury cases and government investigations. That figure represents less than five months of Seroquel sales (Wilson 2017).

APPENDIX G

SSRIS, SEROTONIN SYNDROME AND ALCOHOL

Some of the most commonly prescribed antidepressants are called reuptake inhibitors. What's reuptake? It's the process in which neurotransmitters are naturally reabsorbed back into nerve cells in the brain after they are released to send messages between nerve cells. A reuptake inhibitor prevents this from happening. Instead of getting reabsorbed, the neurotransmitter stays — at least temporarily — in the gap between the nerves, called the synapse (WebMD 2016).

SSRIs cause an influx of serotonin. Alcohol causes a short-lived influx of serotonin. Serotonin Syndrome is caused by too much serotonin building up in the body. Do you see where I am going here?

Check out the conclusion of a study completed in 1997 regarding the role serotonin plays in alcohol abuse:

> Serotonin is an important brain chemical that acts as a neurotransmitter to communicate information among nerve cells. Serotonin's actions have been linked to alcohol's effects on the brain and to alcohol abuse. Alcoholics and experimental animals that consume large quantities of alcohol show evidence of differences in brain serotonin levels compared with nonalcoholics. Both short- and long-term alcohol exposure also affect the serotonin receptors that convert the chemical signal produced by serotonin into functional changes in the signal-receiving cell. Drugs that act on these receptors alter alcohol consumption in both humans and animals. Serotonin, along with other neurotransmitters, also may contribute to alcohol's intoxicating and rewarding effects, and abnormalities in the brain's serotonin system appear to play an important role in the brain processes underlying alcohol abuse (DM 2017).

Alcohol increases serotonin levels in the short term and if you are on a SSRI, it would only make sense that your serotonin levels would skyrocket, sending you into Serotonin Syndrome, where you engage in risky behaviors and act manic. This is also why people would experience "blacking out." The overload sends your nervous system into overdrive. Then, because of the way alcohol works, there is a dramatic drop in serotonin levels, and you would suffer an intensified hangover, one that, if you are already depressed, may cause you to take action when you would not have otherwise.

I think it is fair to say, with such a dramatic fluctuation in serotonin levels, and having hit ecstasy with Serotonin Syndrome, a person might well reach for alcohol when they experience a drop in serotonin levels in order to get back to where they were mentally. In fact, their body may physiologically crave serotonin and cause the person to crave alcohol.

Drug companies would never want drinking to be in the way of their sales, so they don't warn patients in regard to this phenomenon.

> There is an alarming connection between alcoholism and the various prescription drugs that increase serotonin. The most popular of those drugs ARE PROZAC, ZOLOFT, PAXIL, LUVOX, SERZONE, EFFEXOR. For seven years, numerous reports have been made by reformed alcoholics (some of whom have been sober for fifteen years and longer) who feel "driven" to alcohol again after being prescribed one of these drugs. And many other patients who had no previous history of alcoholism have continued to report an "overwhelming compulsion" to drink while using these drugs (Tracy 2017).

Tracy references a scientific study performed in 1994 on a new antidepressant drug, m-Chlorophenylpiperazine [MCPP] that works with the neurotransmitter serotonin. The original study is quoted below:

> m-Chlorophenylpiperazine produced ethanollike effects and alcohol craving in recently detoxified alcoholics... These data further implicate serotonergic systems in the discriminative properties of ethanol and may indicate a serotonergic contribution to craving (Krystal 2017).

APPENDIX H

RX FX: DRUG-INDUCED BLACKOUTS

Throughout high school I blacked out. It became inevitable. No matter what I did, if I drank, at some point of the night, I would lose consciousness mentally, yet appear conscious outwardly.

It was like watching a movie where the film plays without issue right up until a certain point and then the screen suddenly goes completely black: no picture or sound. You wait and wait for the movie to pick back up where it left off, but instead, the film flickers back for a moment, but the scene is blurry, and the characters are now in a completely different time and place than they had been when the screen turned black. Then, before you can sort out what is going on or how the characters got to this new place and time, the screen goes black once more.

Often I would learn that I did mortifying things. It wasn't that I just said embarrassing things, because that is a given drunk-person attribute. I would do things that normal drunk people would never attempt. I heard from different people at various times that at a certain point in the night (usually coinciding with when my memory went dark) my eyes changed. They started to look "vacant."

"You weren't looking back at me. You were, but not really," they would try and explain before shaking their heads. "It was weird; it wasn't you. You didn't look the same."

I attributed these blackouts to the amount of liquor I consumed. And since I don't drink at all anymore, I don't really need to find the answer. But I have strong intuition about this now because many times people did not believe that I had blacked out because they drank just as much as I did or because, they told me, "You didn't even drink that much!" It is very difficult to explain blacking out to a teenager. Most of the time they think you are exaggerating to look cool.

I stumbled across an article about blackouts while researching drug side effects and the definition was spot on for what I experienced countless times.

> A blackout is a period of time where a person is conscious, but is unable to recall any of the events, situations or experiences afterward. A blackout is not passing out, as passing out means you are unconscious. During periods of blackouts, people engage in wild, thoughtless behaviors that they would not typically engage in otherwise (New 2017).

My curiosity, for no specific reason, leads me to search the name of the antidepressant I was taking before the first blackout of this book, alongside the words: "blackout" and "alcohol."

The results are staggering.

I am entranced. I continue down the list of drugs, searching each drug I had been prescribed next to the word "blackouts." I find numerous blog posts of worried individuals wondering if anyone else experiences blackouts while taking [insert antidepressant here] and drinking. Prozac, specifically had over five hundred documented cases of blacking out on one webpage alone (Treato 2016).

Among the list of medications that popped up with significant references to blackouts:

- Prozac
- Lamictal
- Zoloft
- Wellbutrin
- Lyrica
- Effexor

Check out what an attorney says about dealing with his DUI-DWI cases recently:

> As a criminal defense attorney, I see hundreds of clients annually who obtain medications from their physician for anxiety, sleep disorders or depression, yet are not warned to consume NO ALCOHOL when taking these medications. The synergistic effects caused by combining ANY amount of alcohol and these drugs can be devastating for the patient who is surprised to find himself or herself in jail for DUI-DWI, or even vehicular homicide. Blackout, seizures or major amnesia episodes are common. Effexor is currently involved with three of my clients, with others using various common SSRIs and benzodiazepines (Head 2016).

When I tried to find the link that this attorney put in the body of his post, it was broken. I searched the title of his post, "Failure to Warn about SSRIs and Alcohol" and still, nothing. This continually occurred when I tried to access intriguing articles about what patients had experienced while taking certain prescriptions. The links were always broken or the page had been taken down completely.

This happenstance finding of drug-induced blackouts led me to several topics that are truly mind-blowing, including the fact that Serotonin Syndrome actually causes blackouts. And, that blackouts happen in mentally ill people without any substances consumed at all. And the most shocking, that it has been known for a while now that serotonin plays a key role in alcohol craving, dependence and abuse.

It seems pretty obvious to me that if serotonin causes risky behavior and alcohol cravings, it probably causes cravings for other drugs as well. It is like flipping on the switch of addict in individuals who are already weakened by their diagnosed mental disorder. For example, with no history of personal alcoholism or alcoholism in the family, someone taking a serotonergic drug (any of the SSRISs) would be automatically prone to craving alcohol. (See Appendix G.)

APPENDIX I

RX FX NEURONTIN (GABAPENTIN)

- •AED THAT REQUIRES BLACK BOX ON SUICIDALITY

PART A: INCREASED SUICIDALITY

The FDA has completed its analysis of reports of suicidality (suicidal behavior or ideation [thoughts]) from placebo-controlled clinical trials of drugs used to treat epilepsy, psychiatric disorders, and their conditions. Based on the outcome of this review, FDA is requiring that all manufacturers of drugs in this class include a warning in their labeling and develop a medication guide to be provided to patients prescribed these drugs to inform them of the risk of suicidal thoughts or actions. All patients who are currently taking or starting on any antiepileptic drug for any indication should be monitored for notable changes in behavior that could indicate the emergence or worsening of suicidal thoughts or behavior or depression (FDA 2017).

It was after being prescribed Neurontin, that I found myself with a self-proclaimed doctor, who was actually just a drug addict/criminal, at his father's beach house. I'd met him less than two weeks earlier, in an AA meeting.

Shortly after the trip that should have ended in my taking a cab home and blocking Beau's number. I went manic.

One night, I decided I was going to donate all of my things to a second-hand store. I thought Buffalo Exchange was my meal ticket. Everything from UGG boots to True Religion jeans were thrown out of my closet and into a huge pile in the middle of the room. By early morning, I'd gotten through the drawers of my desk and wanted to kill myself amongst the junk strewn around my room. One word: mania. And guess what? Gabapentin was the culprit.

Here a few of the symptoms of depression and/or increased suicidality:

- Talking or thinking about wanting to hurt yourself or end your life.
- Becoming preoccupied with death and dying.
- Becoming depressed or having your depression get worse.
- Withdrawing from friends and family.
- Giving away prized possessions (FDA 2016).

PART B: MANIA

In addition, aside from the usual black-box warning explaining that the medicine your doctor prescribed for your depression causes suicidality, there is also the fact that gabapentin and the withdrawal from antidepressants cause a form of mania referred to as hypomania.

> Several days after the initiation of gabapentin augmentation, Mrs. S reported extreme psychomotor activation, agitation, excessive talkativeness, irritability, insomnia, overspending that was accompanied by writing checks without monies to cover them, and the inability to be 'calmed down.' After two weeks of the preceding symptoms, she was evaluated in an emergency room and treated with oral lorazepam [Ativan]1mg, which was promptly effective for symptom control. Gabapentin was immediately discontinued and the manic symptoms rapidly receded (Sansone 2005).

PART C: HYPONATREMIA

> Hyponatremia has been added as an undesirable effect with unknown frequency to the summary of product characteristics for Neurontin (gabapentin; Pfizer) (The Pharmaceutical 2017).

According to Eric Simon at Medscape, hyponatremia is caused by low sodium in the body and can have fatal effects.

> Symptoms range from nausea and malaise, with mild reduction in the serum sodium, to lethargy, decreased level of consciousness, headache, and (if severe) seizures and coma. Overt neurologic symptoms most often are due to very low serum sodium levels ... resulting in... brain edema (Simon 2016).

PART. D: "ONE OF THE BIGGEST MEDICAL DECEPTIONS IN HISTORY"

> In July, 2003, ... a corporate whistleblower exposed ... Pfizer, 'deliberately distorted information' about Neurontin...putting lives at risk ... in what may be one of the biggest medical deceptions in history.' Pfizer has since been paying heavy fines and settling nationwide lawsuit claims for Warner-Lambert's illegal and deceptive practices (Lawsuits 2017).

After paying huge fines, Pfizer continued to push Neurontin forward.

In 1996, Neurontin started being researched for many off-label uses and has since been aggressively promoted and prescribed for these eleven uses (for which it was not found effective):

- Bipolar disorder
- Pain syndromes, peripheral neuropathy, and diabetic neuropathy
- Treatment of epilepsy alone (as monotherapy)
- Reflex sympathetic dystrophy (RSD)
- Attention deficit disorder (ADD)
- Restless leg syndrome (RLS)
- Trigeminal neuralgia
- Post-hepatic neuralgia (PHN)
- Essential tremor periodic limb movement
- Migraine
- Drug and alcohol withdrawal seizures.

In May 2004, Pfizer paid $430million and pleaded guilty to criminal charges for illegally marketing Neurontin off-label to treat migraine headaches and other pain (Lawsuits 2017).

Neurontin also has an array of mild side effects. A few are listed below:

- decreased coordination
- back and forth eye movements
- persistent sore throat or fever s
- welling of ankles
- mood changes
- memory loss
- or trouble speaking (Lawsuits 2017)

APPENDIX J

BLACK BOX WARNING FOR ANTIEPILEPTIC DRUGS

Like their predecessors, the SSRIs, anticonvulsant drugs all got slapped with a black box warning for suicidality after studies were consistent across the board on eleven different drugs that these medications produce suicidal thoughts.

> AED class label changes: Manufacturers of antiepileptic drugs (AEDs) or anticonvulsant drugs will update product labeling to include a warning about an increased risk of suicidal thoughts or actions and will develop a Medication Guide to help patients understand this risk. The AEDs affected are listed below: Carbatro, Celontin, Depakene, Depakote ER, Depakote sprinkles, Depakote tablets, Dilantin, Equetro, Felbatol, Gabitril, Keppra, Keppra XR, Klonopin, Lamictal, Lyrica, Mysoline, Neurontin, Peganone, Stavzor, Tegretol, Tegretol, XR, Topamax, Tranxene, Tridione, Trileptal, Zarontin, Zonegran (FDA 2017).

Some of the signs of this suicidal behavior include:

- Talking or thinking about wanting to hurt yourself or end your life.
- Becoming preoccupied with death and dying.
- Becoming depressed or having your depression get worse.
- Withdrawing from friends and family.
- Giving away prized possessions (FDA 2017).

APPENDIX K

RX FX: VYVANSE AND ADDERALL

PART A. $56.5-MILLION VIOLATION OF THE FALSE CLAIMS ACT

> Shire Pharmaceuticals LLC will pay $56.5-million to resolve civil allegations ... as a result of its marketing and promotion of several drugs, [Vyvanse, Aderall XR, Dayrana] the Justice Department announced today. ... The settlement resolves allegations that, between January 2004 and December 2007, Shire promoted Adderall XR for for certain uses ... based on unsupported claims that Adderall XR would prevent poor academic performance, loss of employment, criminal behavior, traffic accidents and sexually transmitted disease (The United States Department of Justice [DOJ] 2017).

In addition, Shire allegedly promoted Adderall XR for the treatment of conduct disorder...

> The settlement further resolves allegations that, between February 2007 and September 2010, Shire sales representatives and other agents allegedly made false and misleading statements about the efficacy and 'abuseability' of Vyvanse to state Medicaid formulary committees and to individual physicians ...(DOJ 2017).

APPENDIX L

RX FX: RIFAMPIN (ISONIAZID)

There are reports of total psychosis (Candida 2017) as well as organic brain syndrome or dementia in relation to Rifampin (Pratt 2017). The crazy part is, not only did I hallucinate to the point of terror while trying to sleep and not being able to figure out what was real and what was my brain concocting a very scary world in Beau's bedroom, I was moment to moment unable to remember what I had just done. And the things I did were completely beyond the spectrum of things I would ever, ever do. I remember needing to find a candle and knocking on the neighbor's doors in my pajamas with Beau to find a candle so that I could pray because the hallucinations I was experiencing were utterly terrifying.

> The first three days of treatment ...were uneventful. On the fourth day...the patient suddenly became restless, irritable, and agitated, with aimless, incongruous acts, and irrelevant talking; he also started having visual hallucinations. He had no past history of any mental illness. There was no neurological deficit and fundus examination was normal (as per the neurology evaluation). An initial diagnosis of drug-induced psychosis was made after a psychiatric consultation, with isoniazid Rifampin] being identified as the likely culprit. The patient's symptoms responded to an injection of diazepam (Prasad 2017).

Good thing I carried my own diazepam. Since diazepam seemed to always cure all of my brain issues when I was put on these psychoactive drugs.

APPENDIX M

RX FX: AVELOX, CIPRO, LEVAQUIN, FACTIVE (FLUORO-QUINOLONES)

I got used to feeling bad. Whether it was from starving, medication reactions, or actual illness, I expected to feel loopy, headachy and nauseated. So when I was prescribed antibiotics, especially the big, white Cipro pill, I knew I'd be sick with the same symptoms until I was finished taking them.

Turns out, just this May, a serious FDA Black Box Warning was placed on not only Cipro, but on all fluoroquinolone antibiotics. I knew that a couple of these antibiotics caused everything from hallucinations to night terrors and paranoia in myself. I believed Cipro was a safe one.

Wrong again!

> The U.S. Food and Drug Administration (FDA) approved changes to the labels of fluoroquinolone. "These medicines are associated with disabling and potentially permanent side effects of the tendons, muscles, joints, nerves, and central nervous system that can occur together in the same patient. As a result, we revised the boxed warning, FDA's strongest warning, to address these serious safety issues. We also added a new warning and updated other parts of the drug label, including the patient Medication Guide.
> Patients must contact your health care professional immediately if you experience any serious side effects while taking your fluoroquinolone medicine. Some signs and symptoms of serious side effects include unusual joint or tendon pain, muscle weakness, a 'pins and needles' tingling or pricking sensation, numbness in the arms or legs, confusion, and hallucinations. (FDA 2016)

A few months later, a new statement was released, advising doctors to stay away from prescribing these drugs at all "because the risk of these serious side effects generally outweighs the benefits for patients." (FDA 2016) The reasons for prescribing these drugs include anthrax and plague.

> Because the risk of these serious side effects generally outweighs the benefits for patients with acute bacterial sinusitis, acute exacerbation of chronic bronchitis and uncomplicated urinary tract infections, the FDA has determined that fluoroquinolones should be reserved for use in patients with these conditions who have no

alternative treatment options. For some serious bacterial infections, including anthrax, plague and bacterial pneumonia among others, the benefits of fluoroquinolones outweigh the risks and it is appropriate for them to remain available as a therapeutic option (FDA 2017).

After seven years, on July 25, 2016, the FDA approved the addition of a black box warning for a group of FDA-approved antibiotics (the most commonly prescribed antibiotic in the country) fluoroquinolones. These include; levofloxacin (Levaquin), ciprofloxacin (Cipro), moxifloxacin (Avelox), ofloxacin and gemifloxacin (Factive) (Llamas 2017).

> The labeling changes include an updated boxed warning and revisions to the Warnings and Precautions section of the label about the risk of disabling and potentially irreversible adverse reactions that can occur together (FDA 2017).

This is all well and good. I'm glad there was movement in regard to the study. However, check out how long it took for just a label to be slapped on the medication manual:

- 2008: FDA puts first black box warning on fluoroquinolones for risk of tendinitis and tendon rupture.
- 2011: The risk of worsening symptoms for those with myasthenia gravis was added.
- 2013: Updated label with "irreversible peripheral neuropathy (serious nerve damage."
- 2015: An FDA advisory committee focused on two or more side effects occurring at the same time and causing the potential for irreversible impairment. The advisory committee concluded that the serious risks generally outweighed the benefits…
- July 26, 2016 The FDA approves label changes to enhance warnings about disabling and potentially permanent side effects and to limit use (FDA 2016).

Seven years! And this is the most commonly prescribed type of antibiotic! Seven years was enough time for me to lose my entire young adult and college life, in a trance due to a false diagnosis of symptoms triggered by prescription drugs. Seven years is way too long for 2016. We must change this before it ruins what we have left of the delicate fabric that is humanity.

APPENDIX N

RX FX: ULTRAM (TRAMADOL)

Among the warnings with Ultram are suicide risk, interactions with alcohol, risk of abuse, withdrawal, dependence, interactions with other medications, and it is not to be used for patients who have other "emotional disturbances or depression" (FDA 2017).

> WARNINGS
> Serotonin Syndrome Risk
> The development of a potentially life-threatening serotonin syndrome may occur with use of tramadol products, including ULTRAM ER, particularly with concomitant use of serotonergic drugs such as SSRIs, SNRIs, TCAs, MAOIs and triptans, with drugs which impair metabolism of serotonin (including MAOIs) and with drugs which impair metabolism of tramadol (CYP2D6 and CYP3A4 inhibitors). This may occur within the recommended dose ... Serotonin syndrome may include mental-status changes (e.g., agitation, hallucinations, coma), autonomic instability (e.g., tachycardia, labile blood pressure, hyperthermia), neuromuscular aberrations (e.g., hyperreflexia, incoordination) and/or gastrointestinal symptoms (e.g., nausea, vomiting, diarrhea)" (FDA 2017).

And a new study proves that these ultra-powerful opioid medications, when mixed with benzos become toxic. This is an issue because adolescents or adults either prescribed an opioid medication or taking them illegally, are usually, due to the reason for the pain medication in the first place, people who struggle with anxiety or insomnia. So, if either drug is not reported to their prescribing physician, the two drugs are easily prescribed in tandem by different doctors or used together through different means. The end result can by tragic.

> A [FDA] review has found that the growing combined use of opioid medicines with benzodiazepines or other drugs that depress the central nervous system (CNS) has resulted in serious side effects, including slowed or difficult breathing and deaths. Opioids are used to treat pain and cough; benzodiazepines are used to treat anxiety, insomnia, and seizures. In an effort to decrease the use of opioids and benzodiazepines, or opioids and other CNS

depressants, together, we are adding Boxed Warnings, our strongest warnings, to the drug labeling of prescription opioid pain and prescription opioid cough medicines, and benzodiazepines. (FDA 2017).

APPENDIX O

RX FX: GEODON (ZIPRASIDONE)

This was the second time Dr. Fiaschetti prescribed me Geodon.

Her notes read: "Geodon—worked ok during the summer but in early classes at school, you saw triple. Made you hyper for the 1st three hours after you took it and then groggy all the next day."

In 2007, the FDA attacked Pfizer's Geodon for bad marketing. Pfizer ran an advertisement in a popular medical journal that, according to the FDA was, "false or misleading because it omits important risk information and contains unsubstantiated superiority claims" (Smith 2017). By taking out these risks, the FDA claims that Pfizer "misleadingly suggests that Geodon … is safer than has been demonstrated" (Smith 2017).

Here's some food for thought regarding how big the business of manipulating our mental health has become:

> Geodon sales totaled $400-million in the first half of 2007, according to Pfizer. The drug competes with Johnson & Johnson's Risperdal and Invega, which totaled $2.3-billion in sales during the first six months of 2007, as well as Eli Lilly & Co.'s
> Zyprexa, Bristol Myers Squibb's Abilify
> and AstraZeneca's Seroquel (Smith 2017).

APPENDIX P

RX FX: LAMICTAL (LAMOTRIGINE)

- AED THAT REQUIRES BLACK BOX ON SUICIDALITY

Lamictal is another one of the antiepileptic medications carrying the black box warning regarding its effect and an increase in suicidality (FDA 2009). This is a trend throughout the path of drugs I was prescribed. Here's what the FDA website has to say:

> As described on January 31, 2008, Information for Health Care Professionals Sheet on AEDS, eleven antiepileptic drugs were included in FDA's original pooled analysis of placebo-controlled clinical studies in which these drugs were used to treat epilepsy as well as psychiatric disorders and other conditions. The increased risk of suicidal thoughts or behavior was generally consistent among the eleven drugs … This observation suggests that the risk applies to all antiepileptic drugs used for any indication (FDA 2017).

I hated Lamictal. It was like the Soma for doctors. If there were no solutions, they'd throw in Lamictal. I, however, had to suffer the consequences.

Dr. Fiaschetti's notes read: "at 125mg couldn't get out of bed."

Well, that doesn't work, now does it, Doc?

I felt disconnected from my body on Lamictal: awkward, dizzy, ill. It did nothing for depression. If anything, it worsened depression because I felt so sick and looked so damn pale while taking it!

On Treato.com 375 people posted about taking Lamictal and blacking out. (See Appendix H.) There are posts about waking up being raped, having no control of their body, and blacking out while driving.

APPENDIX Q

RX FX: DEPAKOTE (DIVALPROEX SODIUM)

- AED THAT REQUIRES BLACK BOX ON SUICIDALITY

Depakote is an anti-seizure drug that the FDA also approved to treat bipolar disorder and to prevent migraines. It works by increasing the amount of a special neurotransmitter in the brain, but studies linked its use to suicide, liver toxicity, pancreatitis and birth defects. Its manufacturer Abbott settled a case for $3-million in Arkansas for illegally promoting it to treat schizophrenia and autism, and it settled a $1.5-billion case for illegally promoting it to elderly dementia patients (Drugwatch 2015).

A letter was written to the FDA addressing the concerns about Depakote's serious side effects. Not only is it a dangerous drug without false and misleading marketing, Abbot laboratories, the makers of Depakote were forced by the FDA to correct false and misleading advertisements for Depakote. The statements in the advertisement omitted risk factors, added benefits, and overall, misled the consumer into thinking Depakote ER did something more than its predecessor, Depakote.

> ...it implies that Depakote ER is indicated for use in a broader range of mania patients than Depakote, when this is not the case. Specifically, the Flashcard includes the following claim (emphasis added): 'Expanded acute mania indication with Depakote ER that includes mixed episodes associated with bipolar disorder, with or without psychotic features.' This statement misleadingly suggests that Depakote ER is indicated for a broader mania population than Depakote. In fact, the populations studied in the mania clinical trials of both products were selected using a broad interpretation of acute mania in bipolar disorder, and as described in the PIs for both products, there were no clinical differences between the mania populations studied for each drug (Toscano 2017).

APPENDIX R

RX FX: OPANA (OXYMORPHONE)

Two juvenile females were discovered unresponsive and hypoxic by a male acquaintance. The trio had reportedly crushed and snorted Opana ER tablets and consumed Xanax for recreational purposes. Emergency personnel were able to stabilize one female. The second female was pronounced dead at the scene. ... The cause of death was reported as multiple drug toxicity, and the manner of death was accidental (Vorce 2010).

This is not an isolated issue. As the next article reveals, this is just another story in a bigger web of mass overdoses in juveniles and adolescents and an even larger piece of the opiate addiction epidemic sweeping the United States. (See Appendix W.)

Prescription drug abuse is the new scourge of rural America. It now leads to more deaths in the United States than heroin and cocaine combined, and rural residents are nearly twice as likely to overdose on pills than people in big cities, according to the Centers for Disease Control [CFC] ... At least nine people have died so far this year [2012] from prescription drug overdoses in Scott County, Indiana. Most of the fatalities involved Opana ... Scott County is one of the poorest areas in Indiana ... the drugs cause a vicious cycle of poverty, since abusers cannot hold a job (Wisniewski 2017).

And this epidemic is on the rise; most recently opiate addiction was featured on a major network Primetime news program.

Before 2011, only about 20 percent of the cases referred to the coroner were overdose deaths, and most of those were suicides rather than accidents. Last year, prescription drug overdoses accounted for 19 deaths, or about half of all deaths referred to the coroner in this county of just 24,000 ... Law enforcement officials are alarmed by the rise of Opana abuse, which they said started after Oxycontin was changed in late 2010 to make that drug more difficult to snort or inject for a heroin-like high. Oxycontin is a brand of oxycodone. Opana abuse can be deadly because it is more potent, per milligram, than Oxycontin (Wisniewshi 2017).

APPENDIX S

RX FX: NUVARING

Most birth control pills come with an increased risk for blood clots, but NuvaRing stands out, remarkably because it spiked numbers in healthy twenty-year-olds. These side effects were listed on the NuvaRing website:

- Legs (deep vein thrombosis)
- Lungs (pulmonary embolus)
- Eyes (loss of eyesight.
- Heart (heart attack)
- Brain (stroke) (Merck 2016)

The battle continues with this controversial birth control drug. The FDA had issues approving this drug due to:

> A surprising occurrence that an investigator determined was probably related to the birth control device." This "occurrence" was the development of a blood clot in a previously healthy woman in her 20s (Siddiqui 2017).

I stopped using NuvaRing after my unexplained syncope, or loss of consciousness, behind the wheel and the high-speed three-car crash that took place as a result. This is noted by the neurologist, Dr. Olivera, in my medical charts. Not only did he tell me to stop using NuvaRing, or rather, agreed when I pointed out an article I read about women having strokes out of the blue, he prescribed me Savella. (See Appendix T.)

APPENDIX T

RX FX: SAVELLA (MILNACIPRAN)

PART A. ADVERSE REACTIONS AND WARNINGS

Even the FDA warns against using this drug.

> Savella is not used to treat depression, but it acts like medicines that are used to treat depression (antidepressants) and other psychiatric disorders (FDA 2016).

The adverse reactions are almost endless:

- Serotonin syndrome: agitation, hallucinations, coma or other changes in mental status.
- Seizures or Convulsions.
- Manic episodes reckless behavior, severe trouble sleeping, excessive irritability.
- Visual Problems (Allergen 2017).

These are just a few of the ones listed in Savella's medication manual! These are only the reactions that Allergen was forced to share with the consumer on the package. The actual consumer experiences are horrendous enough to have resulted in a 65,000-person petition written to the FDA to ban Savella completely (Wolfe 2017).

PART B. A PETITION TO BAN SAVELLA

> Margaret Hamburg, M.D., Commissioner
> U.S. Food and Drug Administration
> 5600 Fishers Lane
> Rockville, MD 20857
>
> Dear Dr. Hamburg:
> Public Citizen, representing more than 65,000 consumers nationwide, hereby petitions the Food and Drug Administration (FDA), pursuant to the Federal Food, Drug, and Cosmetic Act 21 U.S.C. Section 355(e)(3), and 21 C.F.R. 10.30, to immediately remove from the market the drug Savella (milnacipran; Cypress Bioscience, Inc. and Forest Laboratories, Inc.) because it has highly questionable clinical efficacy and has been found, in randomized

controlled trials, to cause a large number of potentially serious adverse reactions including hypertension, increased heart rate, and increased suicidal ideation. On July 23, 2009, milnacipran's approval for fibromyalgia was denied in the European Union for these very same efficacy and safety reasons (Wolfe 2017).

The dozen page petition dives into thirteen of Savella's adverse reactions.

It is clear from the list of Warnings and Precautions in the milnacipran label that the use of milnacipran requires both very careful patient selection as well as patient monitoring since some of the adverse effects are life-threatening. The sponsors list thirteen major problems with additional precautions in other sections of the label. We have combined them in the list below:

- Risk of suicide
- Serotonin syndrome
- Increase in blood pressure
- Increase in heart rate
- Increase in seizures
- Hepatotoxicity
- Physical dependence and withdrawal symptoms
- Hyponatremia (low blood sodium)
- Abnormal bleeding
- Activation of mania
- Urethral resistance
- Testicular and ejaculation problems
- Controlled Narrow-Angle Glaucoma: Mydriasis (prolonged dilation of pupil)
- Aggravation of liver disease with alcohol use
- Increased fracture risk
- Hazard to the fetus and newborn
- Hazard to nursing infant
- Risk to those with renal impairment
- Interactions with other drugs
- Gastrointestinal disorders (FDA 2017)

The FDA denied the petition for reasons that don't make themselves clear when reviewing their letter back to Dr. Wolfe.

APPENDIX U

RX FX: NUVIGIL/PROVIGIL (MODAFINIL)

PART A: SIDE EFFECTS

> Confusion about identity, place, and time, hyperventilation and seeing, hearing, or feeling things that are not there (Drugs 2017).

Not even a joke, these are real side effects of taking this drug. I, of course, wasn't warned. Dr. Fiaschetti does not note why I am given Nuvigil. But this is what I found on the FDA website:

> "WARNINGS Psychiatric Symptoms: Post marketing adverse events associated with the use of modafinil have included … aggression (FDA 2017).

I found the piece conveniently replaced by a ellipsis on the FDA website, but present in the required black box warning on the Alembic Pharmaceuticals medication guide:

> Post-marketing adverse reactions associated with the use of modafinil have included mania, delusions, hallucinations, suicidal ideation, and aggression, some resulting in hospitalization. Many, but not all, patients had a prior psychiatric history. One healthy male volunteer developed ideas of reference, paranoid delusions, and auditory hallucinations in association with multiple daily 600 mg doses of modafinil and sleep deprivation. There was no evidence of psychosis 36 hours after drug discontinuation (Alembic 2017).

That's not all, more psychiatric side effects of Nuvigil, which is used in people with excessive sleepiness or narcolepsy, include; "anxiety, agitation, nervousness, irritability and depression" (Alembic 2017). Worse still is the fact that Dr. Fiaschetti either did not know or did not care about the warning regarding taking caution when administering Nuvigil to "patients with a history of psychosis, depression, or mania" (Alembic 2017).

Also, take a look at the mysterious and very profitable acquisition of Cephalon Inc. the designers of the drug. In 2017, I found the same side effects listed on the medication guide but under a new pharmaceutical company, Alembic (Li 2017).

In a first look at modafinil's ascendance on the American pharmaceutical landscape, a group of researchers has shown that use of modafinil grew almost ten-fold between 2002 and 2009, with the steepest rise in uses not approved by the Food and Drug Administration.

> In 2008, Cephalon ... paid $425 million to settle charges that it promoted off-label uses for modafinil and two other drugs. ... Those alleged prohibited promotions may have helped spur the fifteen-fold growth of modafinil prescriptions for off-label uses ... In the same period, prescriptions for patients with diagnoses of narcolepsy, shift-work sleep disorder and sleep apnea grew only threefold. And, one of the steepest jumps ... occurred between 2008 and 2009, after the September 2008 settlement which should have brought a halt to any active off-label promotion (Healy 2017).

PART B: OFF LABEL USES AND A STEADY CLIMB IN CORPORATE AMERICA

> ... almost 90% of patients who were prescribed the medication did not have a diagnosis for which modafinil is an FDA-approved treatment. Patients with depression accounted for 18% of prescriptions; those with multiple sclerosis accounted for 12% ... From 2001 to 2006, the Justice Department said, Cephalon promoted modafinil as a nonstimulant drug to treat "sleepiness, tiredness, decreased activity, lack of energy, and fatigue." The company ignored a 2002 letter and later letters from the FDA ordering it to stop, the Justice Department said (Healy 2017).

The danger comes in using modafinil for the all-too-popular off-label use as this non-stimulant drug to help cognition and brain function after long periods without adequate sleep. Because these drugs were not tested for these uses, the FDA has no reliable studies regarding potentially lethal drug interactions. The clinical trials intentionally left out anyone who was taking an antidepressant or any other medication.

> The clinical trials that led the FDA to approve modafinil specifically excluded potential subjects who were taking antidepressants. The drug's label warns that some patients may have undesired reactions if they take modafinil along with diazepams (such as Xanax or Ativan) or antidepressants. If some of the fastest growth in modefinil use is among those with depression, then potentially harmful drug interactions are likely (Healy 2017).

APPENDIX V

RX FX: ANTABUSE (DISULFIRUM)

- BLACK BOX WARNING FOR COMBINING WITH ALCOHOL

PART A. SIDE EFFECTS

I was prescribed Antabuse because I asked for it by name. I had heard about it in rehab and from my opiate-addicted ex-boyfriend, Jaxx. I was not given any sort of instruction in its use. I was not monitored or told even how many pills to take except for by the label on the actual drug container. I thought it was basically a sugar pill that would make me throw up if I drank, like charcoal or something. Looks like I was far off. Here a few of the listed side effects:

- Confusion
- Unusual thoughts or behavior
- Extreme fatigue or tiredness
- Seizures
- Fainting
- Weakness
- Weak or shallow breathing
- Slow heart rate or weak pulse
- Severe chest pain spreading to your jaw or shoulder
- Loss of appetite
- Upset stomach or vomiting (Epocrates, 2017)

PART B. BLACK BOX WARNINGS

Combining Antabuse with alcohol — such as by taking it while already drunk — can cause a fatal reaction. … Don't take Antabuse if you've consumed alcohol within the past 12 hours. Don't drink alcohol while taking the drug or for up to 14 days after you stop taking it (Epocrates 2017).

I drank while taking Antabuse. It's a drug literally made for alcoholics and addicts, so it would seem pretty reasonable that there would be an issue with this black box warning. It's one thing to be a sugar pill that somehow makes you vomit up all the liquor you drank; it's a whole different horror when this experimentation or simply lack of willpower for just one moment could lead to death. And the patients taking Antabuse usually aren't very stable, since they are taking a medication that solely caters to people who have a pretty bad alcohol problem and need a drug to make them sick if they drink.

For me, in the state I was in and with the brain of lunatic, I thought it was a test to see if anything would happen if I took Antabuse and drank. People actually did this often. And there were a couple times that I had taken Antabuse and just couldn't handle myself and drank late in the night only to get completely plastered and wake up feeling dead.

Jaxx had a prescription too. If we only took one, we would drink anyway and nothing happened until one night he told me the night prior he had more shots than usual on Antabuse and was violently ill. Without his personal experience I would have had no idea it was dangerous. I thought it was a sugar pill.

> Before taking this medicine, tell your doctor if you have, or have ever had:
>
> - Thyroid disease, epilepsy, brain damage or a head injury
> - Mental illness
> - A heart attack or stroke
> - Kidney disease
> - Allergies to medication (Epocrates 2017)

At the time I was prescribed this, I literally had every single one of these issues, including thyroid disease, what was diagnosed as a stroke by the neurologist even though his findings were inconclusive, and documented mental illness. Granted, for me, it was drug-induced, but the records that the doctor who prescribed this to me had, said that I was bipolar, depressed, had fibromyalgia, generalized anxiety disorder, and post traumatic stress disorder. The list goes on and on, but it was well-documented in my medical history. And I know that Dr. Fiaschetti received everything my psychologist in college, Dr. Braun, sent her, because I have the records of them emailing back and forth.

Lastly, of course, I had allergies to medications! The list of my allergies and negative reactions to medications, by this point in 2011, was staggering. Dr. Fiaschetti had all of these at her disposal.

In addition, many common foods and other products might contain a small amount of alcohol that can cause a reaction with Antabuse. These products include:

> - Mouthwash
> - Cough medicines
> - Cooking wine or vinegar
> - Certain desserts
> - Cologne or perfume

- Aftershave
- Antiperspirants
- Antiseptic astringent skin products
- Hair dyes
- Paint thinners, solvents, stains, and lacquers
- Waxes, dyes, resins, and gums (Epocrates 2017)

PART C. LIVER PROBLEMS/FATTY LIVER

You'll need frequent blood tests to check your liver function while taking Antabuse. Be sure to keep all appointments with your doctor and laboratory (Epocrates 2017).

In 2011 an emergency room physician ran some extra tests on me while I was in the emergency room for a kidney infection that had spiked to a high-grade fever. The kidney stone pain had progressed so quickly that within two hours I was in excruciating flank pain again, and running a fever from the Topamax-induced kidney stones I had been passing for years at this point. The doctor told me I had a fatty liver and I was not that concerned because I knew it couldn't be from drinking. But my mom thought otherwise.

APPENDIX W

Rx Fx: Opioids (Vicodin (Acetaminophen/Hydrocodone), Norco (Acetaminophen/Hydrocodone), Roxicodone (Oxycodone), Oxycontin (Oxycodone), Subutex/Suboxone (Buprenorphine)

I always said that these opioid painkillers were an intelligent band of beasts. They attack the brain where it's most vulnerable and with the most addictive qualities. Their name states their effect, but it's bigger than just the physical. They have a physically addictive quality, but they also play mind games with you.

They leave you longing for their familiar haze, years after you've quit. I heard once from a doctor that opiate addiction is the only addiction that stays with you for a lifetime and I completely believe it. I can still taste the chewed-up Norco and the difference in taste when Jaxx switched to Roxis.

They didn't just kill the physical pain. They took the bite out of the everyday. They glossed over the daily redundancies of life. They put a clear, glossy coating over the nails you so carefully painted.

Part A. Vicodin

Vicodin is like a vodka soda, watered down by the ice melting in a steamy club. They were the pills that were stolen from parents' drug cabinets.

Part B. Norco

This has more hydrocodone than Vicodin, but also contains Acetaminophen, Vicodin is child's play in comparison to Norco.

Part C. Roxis

I came to find out that Roxicodone is just a brand name for Oxycodone, which is the same thing as Oxycontin.

Part D. Oxy

80's was the slang term for Oxycontin, which is Oxycodone. No one liked using their actual name, too much bad press, it scared people to say

Oxycontin. For the longest time, nobody touched the drug Oxycontin.

Part E. Subutex

I was taking 80s of Oxycontin while trying to rid myself of the addiction via Subutex and subsequently got addicted to the Subutex, which was given out by my boyfriend, Jaxx, who was going through the same thing only worse.

APPENDIX Y

POST TRAUMATIC STRESS DISORDER

Though only 10 percent of American forces see combat, the U.S. military now has the highest rate of post-traumatic stress disorder in its history (Junger 2017).

A female sufferer who since has recovered from PTSD does a good job at explaining what our body does when it is in constant fear and why:

> From an evolutionary perspective, it's exactly the response you want to have when your life is in danger: you want to be vigilant, you want to react to strange noises, you want to sleep lightly and wake easily, you want to have flashbacks that remind you of the danger, and you want to be, by turns, anxious and depressed. Anxiety keeps you ready to fight, and depression keeps you from being too active and putting yourself at greater risk (Junger 2017).

APPENDIX X

RX FX: SOMA (CARISOPRODOL)

The FDA warns that there have been "post-marketing reports of motor vehicle accidents" (FDA 2017), due to the use of Soma. They also warn, although it is not a controlled substance, that Soma not only produces "withdrawal signs, there are published case reports of dependence," but also "elicits barbiturate-like effects."

And, "in the post-marketing experience with Soma, cases of dependence, withdrawal, and abuse have been reported with prolonged use" (FDA 2017).

Glossary of Useful Terms

AED: Antiepileptic drug

Black Box Warning: A warning placed on a prescription drug label that is encased in a black box outline to call attention to "serious or life-threatening risks" (FDA 2016).

Chronic Stress Syndrome: a complex form of PTSD (post-traumatic stress syndrome).

Hyponatremia: Low sodium in the blood, can be fatal and cause confusion and psychosis.

Interstitial Cystitis (IC): A chronic, painful bladder condition, and as it turned out, a faulty diagnosis for me. I had kidney stones caused by Topamax.

Serotonin Syndrome (SS): "A life-threatening condition caused by having too much Serotonin in the body" (AAFM 2010).

> "This syndrome consists of a combination of mental status changes, neuromuscular hyperactivity, and autonomic hyperactivity. Serotonin Syndrome can occur via the therapeutic use of serotonergic drugs alone, an intentional overdose of serotonergic drugs, or classically, as a result of a complex drug interaction between two serotonergic drugs that work by different mechanisms" (Volpi-Abadi et. al. 2013).

SSRI: Selective Serotonin Reuptake Inhibitors, a type of antidepressant that inhibits the absorption of the neurotransmitter serotonin, e.g. Prozac (Ferguson 2001).

Suicidality: Likelihood of an individual to commit suicide (The Free Dictionary 2016).

References

Alembic Pharmaceuticals. "Modafinil (Alembic Pharmaceuticals Inc.): FDA Package Insert". 2017. *Medlibrary.Org.* http://medlibrary.org/lib/rx/meds/modafinil-22/.

Allergan Pharmaceuticals International Limited. "FDA-Approved Medication Guide MEDICATION GUIDE Savella® (Sa-Vel-La) (Milnacipran Hcl) Tablets." 1st ed. St. Louis: *Forest Pharmaceuticals, Inc*; 2016. Available at: http://www.fda.gov/downloads/Drugs/DrugSafety/ucm089121.pdf.

Alternative to Meds Center. "Lexapro Withdrawal | Alternative to Meds Center." *Alternative To Meds Center.* 2017. https://www.alternativetomeds.com/articles/lexapro-withdrawal/. Accessed July 24, 2016.

American Academy of Family Physicians [AAFP]. "Prevention, Diagnosis, And Management Of Serotonin Syndrome". 2016. Aafp.Org. http://www.aafp.org/afp/2010/0501/p1139.pdf.

Candida, Salafia.. "Rifampicin Induced Flu-Syndrome And Toxic Psychosis. - Pubmed – NCBI".2017. *Ncbi.Nlm.Nih.Gov.* https://www.ncbi.nlm.nih.gov/pubmed/1308530.

Ceasar, Stephen. "Astrazeneca To Pay $68.5 Million In Seroquel Settlement". 2011. *Latimes.* http://articles.latimes.com/2011/mar/11/business/la-fi-0311-astrazeneca-settlement-20110311.

DM, Lovinger. "Serotonin's Role In Alcohol's Effects On The Brain. - Pubmed - NCBI". 2017. Ncbi.Nlm.Nih.Gov. https://www.ncbi.nlm.nih.gov/pubmed/15704346.

Drugs.com. "Ativan: Indications, Side Effects, Warnings - Drugs.Com". 2016. *Drugs.Com.* https://www.drugs.com/cdi/ativan.html.

Drugs.com. "Nuvigil - FDA Prescribing Information, Side Effects And Uses". 2017. *Drugs.Com.* https://www.drugs.com/pro/nuvigil.

Drugs.com. "Nuvigil Side Effects in Detail". *Drugs.com.* 2017. https://www.drugs.com/sfx/nuvigil-side-effects.html.

Drugs.com. "Seroquel - FDA Prescribing Information, Side Effects And Uses". 2017. *Drugs.Com.* https://www.drugs.com/pro/seroquel.html.

Drugs.Com. "Xanax XR - FDA Prescribing Information, Side Effects And Uses". 2016. Drugs.Com. https://www.drugs.com/pro/xanax-xr.html#PRECdi.

Drugwatch. "Prescription Drug Settlement – Litigation For Dangerous Medication". 2016. Drugwatch. https://www.drugwatch.com/prescription-drug-settlements/.

Epocrates. "Antabuse Black Box Warnings - Epocrates Online". 2017. Online.Epocrates.Com. https://online.epocrates.com/drugs/217711/Antabuse/Black-Box-Warnings.

Epocrates. "Opana ER Black Box Warnings - Epocrates Online". 2017. Online.Epocrates.Com. https://online.epocrates.com/u/10b4407/Opana+ER/Black+Box+Warning.

Everydayhealth.com. "Antabuse - Side Effects, Dosage, Interactions | Everyday Health". 2017. Everydayhealth.Com. http://www.everydayhealth.com/drugs/antabuse.

FDA [Food and Drug Administration]. "FDA Drug Safety Communication: FDA Warns About Serious Risks And Death When Combining Opioid Pain Or Cough Medicines With Benzodiazepines; Requires Its Strongest Warning". 2016. Fda.Gov. http://www.fda.gov/Drugs/DrugSafety/ucm518473.htm.

FDA. "FDA Final Response Denying Petition On Milnacipran June 2, 2016". 2017. Citizen.Org. http://www.citizen.org/documents/1900_FDA_Final_Response_Denying_Petition_on_milnacipran_June%203,%202016.pdf.

FDA. "A Guide To Safety Terms At The FDA". 2016. FDA.Gov. http://www.fda.gov/downloads/ForConsumers/ConsumerUpdates/UCM107976.pdf.

FDA. "FDA Drug Safety Communication: FDA reporting mental health drug ziprasidone (Geodon) associated with rare but potentially fatal skin reactions." Fdagov. 2016. Available at: http://www.fda.gov/drugs/drugsafety/ucm426391.htm.

FDA. "FDA Drug Safety Communication: FDA Updates Warnings For Oral And Injectable Fluoroquinolone Antibiotics Due To Disabling Side Effects". 2017. Fda.Gov. http://www.fda.gov/Drugs/DrugSafety/ucm511530.htm.

FDA. "FDA Drug Safety Communication: FDA Warns About Serious Risks And Death When Combining Opioid Pain Or Cough Medicines With Benzodiazepines; Requires Its Strongest Warning". 2017. Fda.Gov. http://www.fda.gov/Drugs/DrugSafety/ucm518473.htm.

FDA. "FDA Public Health Advisory: Suicidal Thoughts And Behavior Antiepileptic Drugs". 2017. Fda.Gov. http://www.fda.gov/Drugs/DrugSafety/PostmarketDrugSafetyInformationforPatientsandProviders/ucm100195.htm.

FDA. "FDA Updates Warnings For Fluoroquinolone Antibiotics". 2017. Fda.Gov. http://www.fda.gov/NewsEvents/Newsroom/PressAnnouncements/ucm513183.htm.

FDA. "Lexapro (escitalopram oxalate) tablets January 2009." Fdagov. 2017. Available at: http://www.fda.gov/Safety/MedWatch/SafetyInformation/Safety-RelatedDrugLabelingChanges/ucm132686.htm\

FDA. "Savella (milnacipran HCl) tablets." Fdagov. 2016. http://www.fda.gov/safety/medwatch/safetyinformation/ucm203615.htm.

FDA. "Seroquel DDMAC Letter – FDA." 2017. Ebook. 1st ed. The Food and Drug Administration [FDA]. http://www.fda.gov/downloads/Drugs/.../UCM221315.pdf.

FDA. "Soma (Carisoprodol)". 2017. *Fda.Gov.* http://www.fda.gov/Safety/MedWatch/SafetyInformation/ucm191961.htm.

FDA. "Suicidal Behavior And Ideation And Antiepileptic Drugs". 2009 Fda.Gov.

http://www.fda.gov/Drugs/DrugSafety/PostmarketDrugSafetyInformationforPatientsandProviders/ucm100190.htm.

FDA. "Ultram ER (Tramadol HCI) Extended-Release Tablets". 2008. Fda.Gov. http://www.fda.gov/Safety/MedWatch/SafetyInformation/Safety-RelatedDrugLabelingChanges/ucm113813.htm.

FDA. "Valium (diazepam) Tablets." Fdagov. 2017. Available at: http://www.fda.gov/safety/medwatch/safetyinformation/ucm374590.htm.

FDA. "Xanax (Alprazolam) And Xanax XR". 2017. Fda.Gov. https://www.fda.gov/Safety/MedWatch/SafetyInformation/ucm271398.htm.

FDA. LEXAPRO™ (Escitalopram Oxalate) - FDA. 1st ed. St. Louis: *Forest Pharmaceuticals, Inc. Subsidiary of Forest Laboratories, Inc.*; 2016. http://www.fda.gov/Safety/MedWatch/SafetyInformation/Safety-RelatedDrugLabelingChanges/ucm132686

Ferguson, James. 2016. "SSRI Antidepressant Medications: Adverse Effects And Tolerability". PubMed Central [PMC]. https://www.ncbi.nlm.nih.gov/pmc/articles/PMC181155/.

Groberman, Alex. "Chronic Stress Disorder". 2017. Psyweb.Com. http://www.psyweb.com/articles/depression/chronic-stress-disorder.

Gupta, Sanjay. 2017. "Unintended Consequences: Painkiller Pills To Heroin - CNN.Com". *CNN*. http://www.cnn.com/2014/08/29/health/gupta-unintended-consequences/.

Head, William C. "Failure To Warn About SSRIs & Alcohol". *Drugs.Com*. https://www.drugs.com/forum/latest-drug-related-news/failure-warn-about-ssris-alcohol-22715.html.

Healy, Melissa. "Use Of Wake-Up Drug Modafinil Takes Off, Spurred By Untested Uses". 2017. LA Times. http://articles.latimes.com/2013/may/02/science/la-sci-stay-awake-drug-modafinil-booming-20130502.

Junger, Sebastian. "How PTSD Became A Problem Far Beyond The Battlefield". 2015. The Hive. http://www.vanityfair.com/news/2015/05/ptsd-war-home-sebastian-junger.

Krystal JH, et al. 2016. "Specificity Of Ethanollike Effects Elicited By Serotonergic And Noradrenergic Mechanisms. - Pubmed - NCBI". Ncbi.Nlm.Nih.Gov. https://www.ncbi.nlm.nih.gov/pubmed/7944878.

Lamb, Tom. "Fibromyalgia Drug Savella Should Be Pulled From Market, Says Public Citizen Group." Drug Injury Watch. 2010. Available at: http://www.drug-injury.com/druginjurycom/2010/01/savella-milnacipran-fibromyalgia-drug-public-citizen-fda- petition-drug-safety.html.

Lawsuits.Lawinfo.com. "Neurontin Lawsuit - Lawinfo". 2017. Lawsuits.Lawinfo.Com. http://lawsuits.lawinfo.com/Neurontin/index.html.

Li, Shan. "Teva, Cephalon: Teva Pharmaceutical Offers $6.8 Billion For Cephalon". 2017. *Latimes*. http://articles.latimes.com/2011/may/03/business/la-fi-teva-cephalon-20110503.

Llamas, Michelle. "FDA Says Risks May Outweigh Benefits for Antibiotics Levaquin, Cipro." *DrugWatch*. 2016. https://www.drugwatch.com/2016/05/16/fda-black-box-warning-for-levaquin-cipro-antibiotic-risk/.

MedFacts, Inc. "Is Serotonin Syndrome A Side Effect Of RIFAMPIN ? (Factmed.Com)". 2017. *Factmed.Com*. http://factmed.com/study-RIFAMPIN-causing-SEROTONIN%20SYNDROME.php.

Merck Pharmaceuticals. "Possible Side Effects of NuvaRing (etonogestrel/ethinyl estradiol vaginal ring)." *Nuvaringcom*. 2016. http://www.nuvaring.com/consumer/risks_side_effects/.

New Life Outlook. "Causes And Treatments Of Bipolar Blackouts". 2016. Newlifeoutlook | Bipolar. http://bipolar.newlifeoutlook.com/bipolar-blackouts/2/.

Oliver, John. 2017. "Opioids: Last Week Tonight With John Oliver (HBO)." Video. https://www.youtube.com/watch?v=5pdPrQFjo2o.

PDR. "Ciprofloxacin Injection | FDA Drug Safety Communication | PDR.net." Pdrnet. 2016. http://www.pdr.net/fda-drug-safety-communication/ciprofloxacin-injection?druglabelid=3255. Accessed July 26, 2016.

PDR. "Neurontin | FDA Drug Safety Communication | PDR.Net". 2016. Pdr.Net. http://www.pdr.net/fda-drug-safety-communication/neurontin?druglabelid=2477.

Physicians Desk Reference [PDR]. "Ativan Tablets (Lorazepam) Dose, Indications, Adverse Effects, Interactions…". 2016. PDR.Net. http://www.pdr.net/drug-summary/Ativan-Tablets-lorazepam-2135.

Prasad, R, Rajiv Garg, and Sanjay Kumar Verma. "Isoniazid- And Ethambutol-Induced Psychosis". 2017. *ncbi.nlm.nih.gov* https://www.ncbi.nlm.nih.gov/pmc/articles/PMC2700450/.

Promises Treatment Center. "Amphetamine's Role In Serotonin Syndrome". 2017. *Drug and Addiction Treatment Centers | Promises*. https://www.promises.com/articles/abused-drugs/amphetamines-role-in-serotonin-syndrome/.

Reuters. "Language Problems Seen With Anti-Migraine Drug". 2017. Reuters. http://www.reuters.com/article/us-anti-migraine-drug-idUSTON60393920080226.

Rottenstein Law Group. "Seroquel Injury Lawsuits: Rottenstein Law Group LLP". 2017. Rotlaw.Com. http://www.rotlaw.com/seroquel/.

Sansone, Lori A. Sansone, Randy A.. 2016. "Hypomania With Gabapentin". Psychiatry (Edgmont) 2 (7): 51. http://www.ncbi.nlm.nih.gov/pmc/articles/PMC3000199/.

Siddiqui, Sabrina. "Side Effects May Include Death." The Huffington Post. 2017. http://www.huffingtonpost.com/2013/12/18/nuvaring-blood-clots_n_4461429.html. Accessed

Simon, Eric. "Hyponatremia." Medscape. 2016. http://emedicine.medscape.com/article/242166-overview#showall.

Smith, Aaron. "FDA Accuses Pfizer Of False Advertising For Geodon - Aug. 13, 2007". 2017. Money.CNN.Com. http://money.cnn.com/2007/08/13/news/companies/geodon/.

Smyres, Kerrie. 2017. "Trouble Thinking On Topamax? Study Finds "Language Disturbances". The Daily Headache.
http://www.thedailyheadache.com/2008/02/trouble-thinking-on-topamax-study-finds-language-disturbances.html.

Sober Living.com. "Spike In Overdoses In Orange County | Sober Living By The Sea, CA". 2017. Soberliving.Com.
http://www.soberliving.com/addiction/opioids/articles/spike-in-overdoses-in-orange-county/.

TH, Pratt. 2017. "Rifampin-Induced Organic Brain Syndrome. - Pubmed - NCBI". *Ncbi.Nlm.Nih.Gov.*
https://www.ncbi.nlm.nih.gov/pubmed/439321.

The Free Dictionary. "Suicidality". 2016. Thefreedictionary.Com.
http://medical-dictionary.thefreedictionary.com/Suicidality.

The Pharmaceutical Journal. "Hyponatremia With Neurontin". 2015. The Pharmaceutical Journal. doi:10.1211/pj.2015.20068524.

The United States Department of Justice [DOJ]. "Shire Pharmaceuticals LLC To Pay $56.5 Million To Resolve False Claims Act Allegations Relating To Drug Marketing And Promotion Practices". 2017. Justice.Gov. https://www.justice.gov/opa/pr/shire-pharmaceuticals-llc-pay-565-million-resolve-false-claims-act-allegations-relating-drug.

Toscano, Amy. "Depakote Letter". FDA.Gov. 2017.
http://www.fda.gov/downloads/Drugs/.../ucm085224.pdf.

Tracy, Ann Blake. "ICFDA Alcohol Cravings Induced Via Serotonin". 2017. Icfda.Drugawareness.Org.
http://icfda.drugawareness.org/Archives/Miscellaneous/MRalcohol.html.

Treato.com "Can Lamictal Cause Blackouts?". 2016. Treato.
https://treato.com/Blackouts,Lamictal/?a=s.

Volpi-Abadie, Jacqueline, Alan David Kaye. "Serotonin Syndrome". 2017. PubMed Central [PMC].
https://www.ncbi.nlm.nih.gov/pmc/articles/PMC3865832/.

Vorce SP, et al. "An Overdose Death Involving The Insufflation Of Extended-Release Oxymorphone Tablets. - Pubmed - NCBI". 2017.

Ncbi.Nlm.Nih.Gov.
https://www.ncbi.nlm.nih.gov/pubmed/21819798.

W., Bill and Bob Smith. 1939. *The Big Book: Alcoholics Anonymous*. 1st ed.

WebMD. "How Different Antidepressants Work". 2016. Webmd.
http://www.webmd.com/depression/how-different-antidepressants-work#1.

Welch, Brian J., Dion Graybeal, Orson W. Moe, Naim M. Maalouf, and Khashayar Sakhaee. 2006. "Biochemical And Stone-Risk Profiles With Topiramate Treatment". American Journal Of Kidney Diseases 48 (4): 555-563. doi:10.1053/j.ajkd.2006.07.003.

Wilson, Duff. 2016. "Astrazeneca Settles Most Seroquel Suits". Prescriptions Blog.
http://prescriptions.blogs.nytimes.com/2011/07/28/astrazeneca-settles-most-seroquel-suits/?_r=1

Wisniewski, Mary. "Painkiller Opana, New Scourge Of Rural America". 2017. Reuters. http://www.reuters.com/article/us-drugs-abuse-opana-idUSBRE82Q04120120327.

Wolfe S, Elisabeth B. "Petition To Ban Milnacipran (Savella)." 1st ed. Public Citizen; 2016. Available at:
http://www.citizen.org/Page.aspx?pid=2596

Thank You

If you enjoyed the book, please share it with your friends! I very much appreciate your support.

Follow me
for updates, giveaways, inspirational posts, and exciting events to come in the
Finding Kali Trilogy!

Twitter: @kaliraewheeler

Instagram: @kaliraewheeler

Blog: kaliraewheeler.com

Do you want to get involved?
Have you been through similar experiences?
Please share!
Help me start the discussion on social media with
#losingkali or #findingkalitriology

I'd love to hear your story.
Or
let's get personal!

Visit kaliraewheeler.com
Click "Connect" & send me a message!

Love and Light <3

Namaste,
Kali Rae Wheeler

www.ingramcontent.com/pod-product-compliance
Lightning Source LLC
Chambersburg PA
CBHW020238030426
42336CB00010B/529